The Heart to Survive

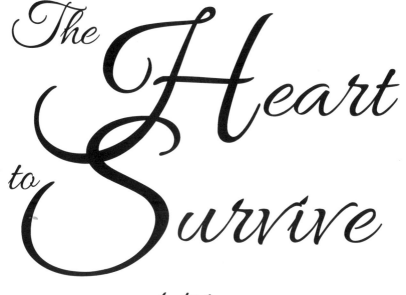

The Heart to Survive

A Memoir

By

Carolyn Powell

in writing collaboration with

Shannon Merillat

Waldman & Company

Minneapolis

This memoir is a work of creative nonfiction. While the events portrayed in this story are true to the best of Carolyn Powell's knowledge, names, places, and other details have been changed to protect the privacy and anonymity of individuals who did not want to be mentioned or whose permissions were either not requested or given. Dialogues may not be exact, as the author may not remember or may not have been present to capture the exact words said by certain people. Since the author seeks to maintain the integrity of events in this case, details have been gathered from people involved to piece together information as accurately as possible.

Published by:
Waldman & Company, Inc., an imprint of

Bookmen Media Group, Inc
331 Main Street South
Rice Lake, WI 54868
www.bookmenmediagroup.com

Ordering Information:
Quantity sales. Special discounts are available on quantity purchases by corporations, associations, and others. For details, contact the publisher at the address above.

Softcover edition ISBN 978-0-9911340-2-1
E-book edition ISBN 978-0-9911340-3-8

Library of Congress
Presassigned Control Number   2014938509

Manufactured in the United States of America
19 18 17 16 15 14 / 7 6 5 4 3 2

Dedication

This book is dedicated to my three favorite boys in my life, Luke, Landon, and Parker. Without all of your continued love and support, I would not be where I am today. It was you that drove me to wake up each day and push myself to get better. You are why I still challenge myself to this day and for that, I am grateful.

I love you, Luke.

I love you, Landon.

I love you, Parker.

Acknowledgements

In the years since my cardiac arrest, I have had a tremendous amount of support from so many people. I am so grateful for my friends, my family, and even the strangers who have given me hope, love, and prayers; visited me in the hospital; and helped care for my two little boys, Landon and Parker. I am blessed to have all of you in my life.

Not only did my friend and former coach, Slade Gormus, offer her encouragement and support to me, but she offered Luke the guidance he so desperately needed in a time that I could not. I am so thankful for Luke's parents (Mike and Debbie, aka Pop-Pop and Dee-Dee), for taking Landon and Parker into their home and giving them love and the guidance they needed. Luke and I are both grateful for this, more than you will ever know!

I would like to thank the paramedics who did not give up on me that night and worked to get my heart started again. Thank you to the emergency room doctors who knew exactly what to do to give me the best chance for survival. The care that I received from the nurses and doctors at both Chippenham Hospital and at the University of Virginia, Health South Rehabilitation Hospital should not go unmentioned. All of my therapists deserve a big recognition for going above and beyond to get me back to where I needed to be to become independent again. Without their dedication and commitment, I would not be where I am today, so thank you!

This book would not have been possible without the work of so many talented and dedicated people. I would like to thank Jaclyn Ruelle for creating the donation website to make this book possible, and everyone who donated and believed in me and my story. I would like to thank Kathi Holmes for her help in the preliminary stages of writing, and Nancy P. Schell, M.D. Board Certified by the American Board of Psychiatry and Neurology, for her contributions; Sue Corns and Dari McDonald at Bookman Media Group, for their guidance, knowledge, and support throughout the whole publishing process. Thank you to Sunshine Urbaniak at Sun Design Studios for developing my website. Thank you to Michelle Graber with Graber's Ink, LLC for her diligent editorial work and for creating the content for my website. And an extra huge thank you to Shannon Merillat for bringing my story to life with her dedication and exceptional writing.

Last, but certainly not least, the biggest thank you I have goes to my best friend and amazing husband, Luke. No matter what the doctors told him, he never gave up on me. He stayed by my side through it all. He tirelessly attended to my every need. To this day, he has never once complained about my disability. He smiles every day and I am so lucky to have such a supportive husband.

Introduction

There are a lot of things I can't do at all anymore, like driving and going for a jog around my neighborhood. That's hard to swallow, being only 32 years old. But there are a lot of things that I can do.

I have to do a lot of things in my own way. It takes me a half hour to pack lunch for my kids, but I can do it.

Five years ago, my heart stopped. I was 27 years old. I had given birth to my youngest son only two months earlier, and my oldest son was just 21 months old. The sudden cardiac arrest I experienced was caused by a chronic genetic heart condition, Long QT Syndrome. The night my heart stopped, my husband found me lying unconscious, with no pulse, next to my oldest son.

It was my oldest son that started the chain of events that made my survival possible. Because of my son's continuous crying, my husband woke up, found me, and called for help. He performed chest compressions until the paramedics arrived. I am alive today because of my son, because of my husband performing CPR, and because of the persistence and expertise of the paramedics, doctors, and nurses at the Chippenham Hospital ER in Richmond, Virginia.

But I'm where I'm at now because of me; because I refused to give up or listen to anyone's expectations. As a result of the cardiac arrest, my brain was deprived of oxygen for a very extended period of time, almost twenty minutes. This oxygen deprivation caused significant brain damage. I had to relearn how to do absolutely everything from the very beginning: how to walk, how to bathe myself, how to write, how to get dressed, how to pick up a slice of pizza, how to give my boys a hug, how to use a fork—among other things.

When I first started walking my son Landon to preschool with my walker, I noticed that the other kids were curious. Some of them had probably never seen a walker before. In 2013, I decided to write a children's book explaining different handicap devices in a way kids could understand, titled *Mommy, What is That For?* When people asked why I wrote it, inevitably my own story would come up. The feedback from everyone was always the same: "That's incredible! You should write a book about your story!"

So I did.

I want to share my story to inspire people to keep going when times are really tough, when all hope seems lost. I want to share what got me through those difficult times. Through my recovery, there were two things that kept me going: taking one day at a time and focusing on the one thing that most motivated me. For me, that one thing was my kids. I wanted to get better so I could be there for them. But that thing could be anything: a loved one, a passion, something you want to accomplish. Anything. You just need to find it, and stay focused on it.

When you have something to focus on, something to work towards, it's easier to not give up. And you can't give up. Even when the doctors—the experts—tell you things are impossible. Not giving up is half the battle. If the paramedics had given up on trying to restart my heart just a minute earlier, I wouldn't be here. But I am here—here to be a mommy for my two sons and here to share my story.

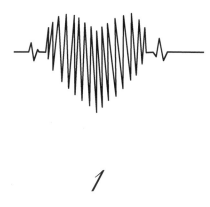

1

The last memory I have before everything happened that evening in July was perfect. My husband Luke, our two little boys, and I were all together as a family, driving back home to Richmond, Virginia, after celebrating the fourth of July at Luke's parents' river house on the Potomac River. As Luke drove across the bridge over the James River, Landon and Parker asleep in their car seats, I remember watching the distant fireworks over Richmond and looking forward to sleeping in my own bed after an eventful weekend away. James Taylor played on the radio. Leaning back, I tousled Landon's strawberry blond hair and gently nudged him, trying to wake him so he could catch a glimpse of the fireworks. He'd never seen fireworks before. But Landon kept on sleeping, worn out like the rest of us.

Almost nodding off to sleep in the passenger seat myself, my thoughts drifted to our upcoming trip to Tampa, Florida. Luke and I would be leaving the boys with his parents while we spent a long weekend in Florida. It would be our first vacation kid-free since Parker was born two months earlier. Like most parents of young children, Luke and I were both in desperate need of some rest and relaxation. The trip was only two weeks away. All the necessary arrangements had been made, our hotel room booked and restaurant reservations made, but we wouldn't end up going. Instead of snorkeling and sipping cold drinks on a beach blanket two weeks after that car trip, I ended up in the Intensive Care Unit (ICU) on life support.

When I awoke from the coma after several days in the ICU, my memory was slow to return. I don't remember anything about the three weeks I spent in the ICU. To tell my story, I have to rely on the memories of Luke, my family and my friends who were there by my side. The first memory I have after my heart stopped beating was inside an ambulance. In that memory, I was being transported from the ICU at the hospital in Richmond to the rehabilitation hospital at the University of Virginia in Charlottesville. Confused and in pain, hot tears streaming down my cheeks, I didn't know what was going on. I didn't understand where I was going. The pain was so bad that the outside world had fallen away. My world then, at that moment, was entirely pain, nothing else.

One other memory I recall of a similar feeling of being very far away and very confused, happened when I was nineteen. I experienced the first symptoms related to Long QT Syndrome when I fainted at Luke's house, while waiting for him to come home from an event for all the basketball coaches at the high school out in Fishersville. We hadn't seen much of each other that week, so we planned on watching a movie and relaxing at his place later that evening. I felt absolutely fine all day. Sometime around 7:30 in the evening, I went to use Luke's bathroom. The last thing I remember before I fainted was walking into the bathroom and shutting the bathroom door.

When I came to, everything looked hazy. I gasped for air. I felt confused. I took in big slow gulps of air, breathing strange, deep breaths. Even though I was breathing heavily, I felt like I couldn't get any air in my lungs. I felt like I was underwater, far below the surface and unable to breathe, with no idea of what direction I needed to swim for air.

I attempted to piece together what was going on: my shoulder pressed up against a wall, and I sat half on, half off of the toilet in what appeared to be Luke's bathroom. I guessed that I must have fainted, but why? I hadn't been feeling ill, and I'd never fainted before. My surroundings offered no clues as to why I fainted.

Fortunately, it seemed that I fainted while seated on the toilet, so I didn't fall. No bruises appeared anywhere I could see, but my energy was completely sapped. I tried to stand up slowly, but I couldn't. My limbs felt like they were made of lead. Slowly, I eased myself down from the toilet on to the floor. Despite hardly being able to breathe, I crawled across the floor to my cell phone, in the adjoining bedroom on Luke's dresser. Crawling this short distance left me dripping with sweat and utterly exhausted—like I'd been running a marathon in the middle of August. I fumbled with the buttons on the phone for a few minutes, trying to remember Luke's cell phone number. I racked my brain, but the numbers wouldn't come to me. My thoughts were too scattered and fuzzy. Finally, I managed to remember the speed dial for Luke's cell phone. After a few tries, I hit the right button. A few rings later, Luke answered and said he'd be here in a few minutes.

I was so hot! Thinking fresh air might help, I crawled out into the front yard to wait for Luke. I laid on my back in the cool grass, staring up at the darkening late evening sky. The sun had set, but the western edge of the sky glowed gold. Coupled with the cool November air, the damp grass felt good and cool against my hot skin, but I still felt feverish and sweaty. More confused than anxious, I wondered, *what is happening to me?* I was young and healthy. At nineteen years old, having spent nearly my whole life playing sports and eating well, my body was in nearly perfect physical condition. This didn't make any sense.

Luke arrived within minutes of my call and drove me straight to the emergency room. The doctor took my blood pressure and asked me the usual questions about my medical history. The doctor said it was a good thing I'd made it to the hospital when I did; my blood pressure was dangerously low: 76/40. My blood pressure caused my body to go into shock. When I say shock, I don't mean I was in an emotional state of shock. I wasn't surprised or upset or anything. Shock is actually a condition that happens when a person's blood pressure drops so slow that not enough blood gets to the brain and other organs. When the brain and other organs do not receive enough blood, they eventually stop working, and when organs stop working, death quickly follows. In other words, shock is quickly fatal, if left untreated. I almost died.

The doctor treated the low blood pressure right away. A nurse gave me fluids through an IV to increase my blood volume. Luke sat with me while I waited for my blood pressure to return to normal. Slowly, I began to feel a little better. I didn't feel like I was drowning underwater anymore, but I still felt totally exhausted.

The doctor wanted to find out if my fainting spell was a result of a heart condition, so he ordered an electrocardiogram, also known as an EKG. The technicians took me into another room in a wheelchair. Luke came with me. I had never had an EKG before, but it was painless. The technicians stuck a few sticky electrodes underneath my hospital gown to different spots on my chest.

The low blood pressure was easy enough to fix, but it turned out the underlying cause was not. After reading the EKG, the doctor diagnosed me with Long QT Syndrome. He gave me a brief and matter-of-fact description of my condition: Long QT Syndrome is a heart condition where there is a disturbance in the heart's electrical system. This glitch in the electrical system of the heart can cause the heart to beat irregularly. This abnormal heart rhythm is called an arrhythmia. An arrhythmia caused by Long QT Syndrome caused my blood pressure to suddenly drop.

Long QT Syndrome is chronic, so it wasn't going to go away; I'd have to deal with it for the rest of my life. The condition is typically managed with medication or sometimes an implanted device, like a pacemaker or an internal defibrillator, he said. Lifestyle changes, like avoiding certain kinds of exercise and physical activity, are often necessary.

The doctor recommended that I also follow up with a cardiologist immediately. I didn't need convincing. This sounded serious. I wanted to get this under control right away. I was concerned, but I thought *I will just get this sorted out now, so that everything can go back to normal.* That's how I always approached challenges throughout my life— directly and quickly. It was how I passed anatomy class in college and mastered lifts in synchronised swimming routines. Up until my sudden cardiac arrest a few years later, this approach had been very effective.

I planned on making an appointment with a

cardiologist the following day for some time later in the week after class. When I left the hospital, my mind felt much clearer. I didn't feel feverish anymore, but I still felt exhausted. When I got home from the emergency room that evening, I did what most people newly diagnosed with an unfamiliar medical condition do: I Googled it.

Suffice it to say I was more than a little unsettled to find that sudden death was one of the most common symptoms. I read somewhere that the cardiac arrhythmias Long QT Syndrome can cause are the most common cause of sudden death in people under thirty. Normally I would've found all of this medical information fascinating. On any other day, I would've been genuinely interested in the descriptions detailing what part of the heart was responsible for an arrhythmia, but that night, all I could think about was the prospect of sudden death. I had a condition where I could just fall over dead for no reason, at any time. I was scared. Making an appointment with a cardiologist couldn't wait until later in the week.

The next day, I skipped class and drove all the way to Richmond from Harrisonburg for an appointment I'd scheduled with Dr. Carter, a cardiologist.

Dr. Carter gave me a more detailed description of Long QT Syndrome. Combined with the research I did myself soon after I was diagnosed, I became pretty knowledgeable about my condition. Initially, I found it easier to understand Long QT Syndrome in terms of what it looks like on a heart monitor. The heart monitor works by recording the electrical activity of the heart. The information about the heart's electrical activity is shown on a graph, displayed on a monitor. The graph looks like a horizontal line with sharp peaks and valleys. The peaks and valleys represent the electrical activity happening when the heart beats. Electricity is what makes the heart beat. Carefully regulated electrical signals cause the walls of the heart to contract and pump blood to the rest of the body.

Each heartbeat is actually a complex process, involving a series of precisely timed events. Within each heartbeat, there are five different electrical waves that can be seen on an EKG. They are each given letters: P, Q, R, S, and T. Normally, the interval between the Q and T waves—the QT interval—accounts for a third of the total time of each heartbeat. In Long QT Syndrome, the QT interval lasts longer than normal. So, the name of the condition is pretty straightforward: people that have Long QT Syndrome have a long QT wave on the EKG.

The heartbeat of someone who has Long QT Syndrome is always abnormal. The QT interval lasts too long in each heartbeat. Most of the time, the pattern that can be seen on an EKG is consistent, and the heart is able to effectively pump blood to the body's organs. The problem is that this abnormal heartbeat, this prolonged length of time between the Q and the T wave, can lead to a sudden upset in the precise timing of electrical impulses involved in each heartbeat. It's precise down to the millisecond, and if the timing is just a little bit off, the heart can't correctly reset itself and recharge like it should.

This short-circuiting of the heart can cause a sudden and dangerous arrhythmia. Often, there are no symptoms before one of these arrhythmias. It was one of these dangerous arrhythmias that caused both my first fainting spell I had at nineteen when I was waiting for Luke to come home from the basketball coaching event, and the life-altering sudden cardiac arrest that I experienced years later. In both of these cardiac episodes, the timing of the electrical impulses went awry, and my heart started to beat out of control. When the heart's electrical signal short-circuits, the heart fails to reset itself and quivers instead of contracting. This quivering motion does not effectively pump blood to the rest of the body. When I fainted in Luke's apartment, the arrhythmia did not last. My heart was able to correct itself. It slowed down, and regained its normal rhythm. Years later when my heart stopped, the arrhythmia was so severe that my heart couldn't fix it. And it wasn't clear right away if it could be fixed at all by anything.

I expected an elaborate plan of attack that included undergoing surgery, getting a pacemaker, taking lots of medication, and making other drastic changes to my daily routine. Actually, I *hoped* for an aggressive treatment plan to follow. I think it would've made me feel a little more in control of my condition; a condition that threatened to take away what control I had over my own health. What I found especially unsettling about this condition was that no matter how healthy I ate or how much I exercised, sudden death was still a significant risk. To my surprise, Dr. Carter only gave me a prescription for a beta-blocker—a type of drug that slows the heart rate and has been shown to be effective at preventing dangerous arrhythmias. One pill a day, and that was it.

Dr. Carter recommended that I make a follow

up appointment for three months later, but easily reassured me that I would be "fine, just fine."

"You have nothing to worry about. You are young, healthy, and athletic. True, you have a heart condition, but it is a minor one. Statistically speaking, you'd be more likely to die getting struck by lightning," Dr. Carter smiled warmly.

"Still," I asked him, "Are you sure I shouldn't get a pacemaker? Just as a precaution? Against, you know, sudden death?" No?

"How about an internal defibrillator?"

No.

I felt like I should be doing much more. I wanted to be doing much more. Dr. Carter explained that a pacemaker, or any treatment besides the beta-blockers, was simply unnecessary; besides the recent fainting episode, I hadn't experienced any symptoms at all. The majority of people who have Long QT Syndrome live long, full lives and never experience dangerous arrhythmias.

Dr. Carter said "The QT interval only appeared mildly prolonged on the EKG, so you don't need to worry."

Easier said than done.

After that first visit to the cardiologist, I still felt shaken. For the next week, I continued to research Long QT Syndrome. What I found mostly confirmed what my cardiologist said—sporadic mild symptoms like mine didn't necessitate medical intervention beyond beta-blockers. I had done all of the recommended diagnostic tests: I had an EKG done, I completed a stress test, and I wore a Holter Monitor for a week following my first cardiologist appointment. A Holter Monitor is a small portable heart monitor, about the size of a cell phone, with several wires that attach to your chest. It shows any possible variation in the QT interval—whether or not it was ever more than mildly prolonged. It can also detect and document any arrhythmia that might occur while I was wearing it. There was nothing.

About two years later, during my internship as a registered dietician at the University of Virginia in Charlottesville, I made an appointment to visit one of the doctors that came to the University to lecture, Dr. Andrews. I could tell from his lecture that he was on top of the latest research and treatments. Dr. Andrews did another EKG, which confirmed my heart's mildly prolonged QT wave. He suggested a stress test might reveal some valuable information about how Long QT Syndrome was affecting my heart and my body. So, we scheduled one.

For the stress test, the technicians attached all kinds of wires to my skin. Dr. Andrews monitored the information the wires transmitted back to the machine while I walked on a treadmill. Every few minutes one of the technicians increased both the incline and the speed of the treadmill. This went on for about thirty minutes. Throughout, Dr. Andrews stood close by and discussed the readings with me. He kept mentioning what outstanding physical condition I was in. Besides the long QT wave, my heart appeared strong and healthy.

After a four-minute interval of running at a pretty good clip, Dr. Andrews shook his head. "You are clearly an athlete!" he said.

I smiled a little and said, "Yep, I sure am!"

Because of the results of the EKG and the stress test, Dr. Andrews didn't see any need to alter my treatment. Beta-blockers would be sufficient to treat my mild Long QT Syndrome. Again, I asked about having a pacemaker implanted. Again, I was told that would not be necessary. This time, my fears had been quieted. My heart was strong; my Long QT Syndrome was mild; and multiple cardiologists were confident that my life was not in danger.

Looking back on all this years later, I want to say that my cardiologists did everything right. At the time I was diagnosed, doctors really didn't know very much about Long QT Syndrome. They didn't know how serious it was. They didn't know how common sudden cardiac arrest was in patients that had only mild, infrequent symptoms. Doctors didn't yet know that sudden death was frequently the very first symptom of Long QT Syndrome. Even now, much less is known about Long QT Syndrome compared to other heart conditions. Today, almost fifteen years after I was diagnosed, treatment tends to be more aggressive.

Over the next few years, apart from experiencing dizzy spells if I stood up too quickly, I felt fine. It's likely the dizzy spells were caused by my low blood pressure, which had nothing to do with Long QT Syndrome. Years passed, and Long QT Syndrome faded away into the background. It seemed it wasn't actually the life altering condition I thought that it would be when I was initially diagnosed. Long QT Syndrome had almost no presence in my daily life. It wasn't something I thought much about. I took my beta-blocker every day, but my daily life went on as usual. I brought it up if I saw a new doctor and included it in the medical history section of various forms I encountered over the years, but that was it. Even when I was pregnant with both of my children, Landon and Parker, I didn't have any other symptoms. Both were easy pregnancies with no complications of any kind.

It wasn't until seven years after I was diagnosed that I experienced any symptoms worth noting. Unfortunately, that first symptom that I experienced after those seven years was sudden cardiac arrest.

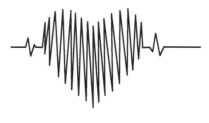

2

For a while, I wanted to name our second son Hudson. During my sixth month of pregnancy, in January of 2009, "Hudson" got stuck in my head. The news constantly aired the name—on January 15th, a commercial plane had taken off from New York City and lost power in both engines shortly after colliding with a flock of Canadian geese only minutes into the flight. With not enough time to get to a runway, the pilot emergency landed in the Hudson River. The news reported minor injuries, but all 155 of the passengers and the crew survived. Everyone called it the "Miracle on the Hudson." Hudson. I liked the way the name sounded, and I liked that it was associated with a miracle.

Before the Miracle on the Hudson happened, both Luke and I liked the name Parker best. Luke wasn't a fan of Hudson. He remained set on Parker, and it was my second choice, so that's what we named him: Parker Wade Powell.

I consider both of my sons to be miracles in the same way that all babies are miracles, but there wasn't anything miraculous about the way they came into the world. My pregnancies with both were a breeze. I took some time off from running, but I still exercised and still ran around in high heels during the entire nine months.

Until the summer of 2009, I really hadn't encountered any sort of miracles first hand. I saw them on the news and talk shows, and I read about them in magazines. But besides my baby boys, nothing truly miraculous had ever actually happened to me. That would change the night of July 5th. A few weeks after that night, the fact that I was even alive was a miracle.

Up until I gave birth to Parker, I worked as a registered dietician at the University of Richmond. I'd been there since 2005, right after I finished up my internship at the University of Virginia in Charlottesville. After Parker was born, the plan was to go back to work part-time in the fall. I had worked out a plan for going back to work part-time, three days a week. We had a babysitter lined up to come to the house and look after the boys one day, and Luke's mom, Debbie, was going to watch them the remaining two days. I felt like I had a pretty good work/life balance going on. I spent time with my sons and my husband, exercised every day, and pursued a career I loved. And to me, that's exactly what being a super mom is all about: successfully balancing work life and family life.

Growing up, I wanted to be a doctor. As I got older, I started to reconsider. Ten more years of school after high school? Thanks, but no thanks. But I still wanted to pursue a career in health care. The fast-paced nature of the field enticed me, and I loved working with people.

I considered being a dietician as a career option in high school, when a friend showed me the food journal her dietician told her to keep. She worked with a dietician as part of her treatment for an eating disorder. In the journal, she recorded what she ate, how much she ate, and how she felt after eating it—anxious, calm, happy, sad, etc.

At my urging, she explained to me how exactly her dietician helped her. Her dietician helped her explore her relationship with food. She helped her figure out what foods and how much of them she needed to eat to be healthy. I found all this fascinating. When I looked into it on my own, I learned that being a dietician also involves a lot of planning—planning out meals for patients to fit their unique dietary needs and their lifestyles. So it seemed that this career was the intersection of one of my biggest strengths and two of my biggest interests: planning, food, and exercise. When I took my first nutrition class in college, I was hooked. I'd found my calling.

At the University of Richmond, I worked with students, faculty, and staff—but mostly students—helping them to manage their weight and keep to special diets. My clients had a wide variety of needs. I helped football players wanting to gain weight, I helped people who were overweight and wanting to lose weight, I helped people overcoming eating disorders, I helped people dealing with food allergies, and I helped people who were trying to manage certain chronic health conditions, like diabetes. I loved guiding them—helping them get healthy and achieve their goals—and I loved seeing the results.

In the weeks before my heart stopped in the summer of 2009, I felt like I was living the dream. I had given birth to my second son, Parker, on Easter Sunday. We had a home of our own in the south side of Richmond, Virginia, not far from where

I'd grown up. I had a loving family of my own, a job I loved, and a home I loved. It was perfect. Everything seemed to be falling into place.

Not only did I have everything I'd ever really wanted in life—a loving husband, two kids, and a great job—I felt like a supermom. I felt like I had it all, and I was doing it all. The summer of 2009 was hectic, but I successfully juggled everything. And with Luke travelling more and more for work, there was more and more for me to juggle. Luke worked as a sales rep for General Electric in Richmond. The timing was not the best, but he and I both knew when he started with General Electric a few years ago that, at some point, he would need to start travelling a lot for work. I knew it was going to be a challenge, but I could handle both boys on my own, no problem. Having Luke gone more often just meant that I'd need to do a little more planning, which was not a problem for me.

I was grateful for everything I had, except for one thing. It was something that I had always had, which is probably why I didn't think about it. It was something that I was incredibly fortunate to have: my health.

I knew I had a heart condition, but I'd been assured by all of my doctors that it was minor. The initial diagnosis of Long QT Syndrome when I was nineteen—after the fainting episode that landed me in the emergency room—was really the only deviation from a lifetime of good health that I ever experienced. In the summer before my cardiac arrest, I felt great. My pregnancy with Parker had been just as easy as my pregnancy with Landon. I was back to running every morning with the boys in the jogging stroller just three weeks after Parker was born.

As a dietician, I practiced what I preached: healthy eating and regular exercise. But these things were second nature. When I was growing up, my mom practiced a very healthy lifestyle, going to the local fitness center often. She was a great role model, and I followed her example early on. I had my vices, namely candy, but I've always preferred humus and veggies to potato chips. I never really thought much about my health, because I didn't have to. I thought about the things I needed to do to be healthy, but I didn't actually think about my health. I didn't realize how lucky I was. There are lots of people that have extremely healthy lifestyles and still struggle with all kinds of diseases and health problems. I know many of my clients did. I took my good health for granted. Without it, as I would soon find out, doing all of the things that I loved would be almost impossible.

Life became especially busy after Parker was born, so I was happy for the opportunity to relax at the river house over the Fourth of July weekend. The river house, on the outskirts of Montross, Virginia, was along the Potomac River, between Ragged Point Beach and Nomini Bay. The Potomac feeds into the Chesapeake Bay not far from there. It's quiet, when there aren't fifteen other relatives there with us, but even then it still feels peaceful. Water, be it a lake, a river, or an ocean, has always brought me peace.

The river house belongs to Luke's parents. They bought the property when Luke was in high school. Luke's mom and dad, Mike and Debbie, built the house a few years later—a cozy house on thick, sturdy wooden stilts. The house always reminded me of a tree house, probably because of the stilts. There's a wrap-around porch that stretches around the front, and a tiny wrought iron weather vane perched on top. In the summer, the tables on the porch were usually all covered in brown paper for putting the crabs on. We would order crabs from a local seafood market. Fond memories of feasting on all that crab on the front porch overlooking the river, and especially of that Fourth of July weekend, remain. That was Landon's first time eating crab, and he loved it.

Once we arrived at the river house we could relax, but getting everything ready to go could be a challenge. Going anywhere with a baby and a toddler requires a lot of planning. Whenever we went to the river house, I always wrote out a detailed list of things to pack in my notebook, only checking each item off when it was actually safely packed and ready to go. Because the river house is so remote and it's a trek to get to even the closest store, I had to make sure we had everything we could possibly need for the weekend: two different sizes of diapers, baby formula, distilled water, Tylenol in case either kid got a fever, extra pacifiers…the list of things to pack was extensive.

That weekend at the river house, I spent most of my time sunbathing and napping in the hammock on the front porch with Parker snuggled up on my chest. Occasionally, I'd join one of the ongoing games of croquet in the side yard. It was as relaxing as can be for a mother of two young boys. I had to make sure someone watched Landon at all times. He'd disappeared earlier in the summer at our house in Richmond.

Our backyard at home was fenced in, so I let Landon play in our backyard there while I did laundry or made dinner, always listening and peeking out the window now and again to make sure he was okay. He liked to play with his little basketball and his Little Tikes® kid-size basketball hoop. I could usually hear him dribbling his basketball, but one afternoon the dribbling stopped for a few minutes and didn't start again. I heard nothing but unbroken silence in the backyard. I looked out the window: no Landon. I poked my head out the back door: no Landon. Panicked, I searched the backyard. The gate to the front yard was open, and there was no Landon in sight. On my way to check upstairs before I set off to search the neighborhood, I caught a glimpse out the front window of a little boy dribbling a basketball across the street. It was Landon, thank God.

I worried about my children running away or getting hurt, but it never crossed my mind to worry about them losing me, their mother. Why would it? I always tried to plan ahead and be ready for the unexpected, but I was healthy and young. At the time, I thought that wouldn't be something I would need to think about until I was much older, after Landon and Parker were grown.

Keeping track of Landon at the river house was not an easy task. He was all over the place, running around the grass in his diaper, splashing around in the kiddie pool, playing with his trains in the shade underneath the house, and following his Pop-Pop (Luke's dad) around. At the age of two, Landon's energy seemed endless. Landon took to following Pop-Pop around during our weekend at the river house and loudly announcing that he wanted to go for a boat ride, shouting "Boat! Boat!" Landon kept attempting to lead Pop-Pop over towards the dock. When Luke and his father finally succumbed to Landon's wishes, securing Landon in his little life vest, Landon immediately fell asleep in Luke's arms. The soothing lapping sound and the rhythm of the water was just too much for the little guy.

A day before we left for the river house, my mom came by our house in Richmond to bring over an inflatable kiddie pool for Landon. While we were in the yard setting it up, she stopped and looked at me for a moment. I could tell she was really concerned about something.

"Carolyn," she said, "you look so tired. You look absolutely exhausted! Are you feeling okay?"

I laughed, rolling my eyes a little. "Mom, I've got two babies, both under the age of two. Of course

I look tired. Welcome to mommy-hood, right?" I thought it was strange that she was so concerned, but I shrugged it off. I didn't feel any more tired than I normally did, getting up at least twice during the night with the boys.

I hardly ever take "selfies," but for whatever reason, I took one of Parker and me snuggling at the River House that weekend. I posted it on Facebook the day we came back home from the long weekend. That was the same day my heart stopped. I don't even remember taking that photo, much less why I took it. I can only guess that I took it in the morning—I'm not wearing any make-up, and my brown hair is pulled back in a messy ponytail— you can't see that it's curly in the picture. Parker is wearing a yellow t-shirt that was a little too big for him. I'm smiling at the camera, my big brown eyes are looking straight at the lens, and Parker is looking down in the way that babies do, not able to really focus. It was a moment that at the time seemed so ordinary, something easily taken for granted. When I snapped that photo, I had no idea that it could easily have been the very last photo of me with Parker.

Fortunately, it wasn't the last picture of me with Parker. It was the last picture that I took myself for a while, but it wasn't the last one. And for that I'm eternally grateful.

My dad took the next photograph of Parker and me together, about two months later. It's similar to the one of us snuggling at the river house: Parker isn't looking at the camera; I'm not wearing make-up; and my hair is tied back. The main difference is that in this photo, I'm in a hospital room, sitting in a wheelchair, hospital ID bracelet on my wrist. Parker is sitting in my lap, wearing adorable little corduroy overalls and a stripped long sleeve shirt. In the picture, it looks like I'm holding Parker. He's on my lap and my arms are around him, but Luke positioned my arms like that—not me. At the time, my arms were too weak and spastic to actually hold either Parker or Landon.

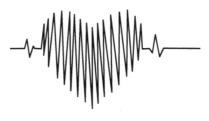

3

After we all went to bed on Sunday, July 5th, I woke up to Landon crying in the middle of the night. As usual, I got out of bed quickly and padded down the hall the short distance to his room.

When Luke found me about ten minutes later, I was curled up next to Landon in his bed. The wooden rails along the sides of Landon's bed made getting in and out of his bed difficult for anyone besides a small child. So instead of getting in bed with Landon when he woke up crying, I normally knelt beside his bed to calm him. Landon seldom slept through the night, so I was up with him most nights. On nights when I knelt beside him, I gently ran my hand up and down Landon's back, talking softly to him, telling him there was nothing to be scared of, everything was okay. Sometimes I picked him up and rocked him, holding him so his head rested on my chest. If he was particularly upset and crying a lot, his tears would leave little cold, damp spots on my t-shirt.

I think I maybe felt slightly dizzy after I got up, but dizziness had never been an issue before. So I didn't notice anything strange about the way I felt that night. And this certainly wasn't the first time that I'd been abruptly woken up in the middle of the night by a crying baby. That night, I think I must have gotten into bed next to him just because I was so exhausted from the long holiday weekend, thinking I could at least rest my eyes while I calmed him down. My heart probably stopped after I lay down with Landon. If I had fainted, there's no way I would've collapsed so neatly.

As I lay still and lifeless beside my son, Landon kept crying. Luke woke up. Hearing Landon crying and seeing me gone from bed, Luke called out to ask if everything was okay. No answer. The whole house was silent, except for Landon. At this point, Landon's cries had turned to shrieks. Luke called out again. Still, no response. Sensing something wasn't quite right, Luke hurried to Landon's room and snapped on the light: Landon was sitting up in bed crying, my body lying next to him, my skin pale and starting to tinge purple.

Luke immediately knew I needed help. Although he wasn't sure exactly what had happened, Luke sprang into action. He did all of the things that people are supposed to do in a medical emergency.

Luke tried to shake me awake. I didn't stir. Luke ran to the other room and grabbed the phone to call 911. When he returned to Landon's room, Luke could tell I wasn't breathing. He checked my pulse. There was none. My heart had stopped beating. Luke lifted me from the bed and gently placed my body onto the floor, where he set to work performing CPR on me until help arrived.

A few minutes after Luke called 911, an ambulance pulled into the driveway, sirens blaring. Luke ran downstairs to open the door for the paramedics, after the dispatcher on the phone told him the ambulance had arrived. Still only wearing his boxer shorts, Luke ushered the paramedics to the stairway and pointed them to Landon's bedroom. The two paramedics climbed the stairs with the gurney, Luke trailing behind them. Right away, the paramedics took out the defibrillator and started trying to restart my heart.

"Get the kid out! Get the kid out of the room now!" One of the paramedics barked.

Landon was still sitting up in bed and crying.

Somehow still clear headed, Luke scooped up Landon and left the room. Luke settled Landon into our bed in our bedroom. Then, Luke turned the bedroom TV on and switched the channel to cartoons in order to settle Landon down and drown out the chaos—Luke hoped to provide Landon with some sense of normalcy.

Next, Luke called his parents. "Carolyn passed out, and she's being taken to the hospital, and you need to come over and watch the boys," he told his mom.

Nearly five minutes had passed since the paramedics started trying to shock me back to life. Nothing. The paramedics continued trying to restart my heart. Luke could hear them shouting.

"Clear!"

"Charging."

"Clear!"

"Charging."

"Clear!"

Parker woke up crying. Luke made him a bottle amidst the increasing chaos. Luke later told me that as he was feeding Parker, several more paramedics and police officers materialized in the house. The ambulance, the fire truck, and three police cars parked out front illuminated the entire street with flashing red and blue lights. A small group of neighbors had gathered across the street, but they kept their distance. Luke continued to try to keep the boys calm, all the while keeping tabs on what the paramedics were saying and what was going on.

Death or permanent brain damage is likely to occur within four to six minutes of cardiac arrest. If a cardiac arrest lasts longer than ten minutes, survival is rare. Extremely rare. Lasting irreparable brain damage is almost certain to occur if the heart isn't restarted within this amount of time. The paramedics had been trying to restart my heart for almost ten minutes. My heart had stopped ten minutes before they had arrived, which meant my heart had not been beating for twenty minutes.

At that point, one of the paramedics approached Luke and asked how long I had been unconscious. Luke told him what time he found me and how much time he had spent performing CPR on me. The paramedic nodded and told him things weren't looking good for me. Luke was worried when he heard this, but the reality didn't fully sink in. Maybe it was the adrenaline that made him unassailable. Luke is generally good at dealing with emergencies. He just does whatever needs to get done. If you asked Luke for advice on how to handle tough situations, he'd probably tell you, "Take one thing at a time, and just go forward." I would probably tell you the same thing, because I'm the same way.

Just as the paramedics were beginning to lose hope, my heart started beating again. Within seconds, the paramedics loaded me on the gurney and carried me down the stairs to the ambulance. Mike and Debbie (Luke's parents) arrived at the house to look after Landon and Parker, just as the ambulance pulled away. A police officer offered to drive Luke to the hospital. From the backseat, Luke started making phone calls to my family. He said the hardest call to make was to my father. Luke's hands were shaking when he dialled the number. Hardly anyone answered, because it was so late at night. Luke left messages, saying the same thing he'd told his mother: that I had passed out and was being taken to the hospital.

At the hospital, the doctors hooked me up to life support machines. Doctors and nurses quickly prepared an ice bed for me. Using therapeutic hypothermia, the doctors tried to cool my body to prevent potential brain damage. My body temperature cooled for twenty-four hours. The next forty-eight hours were spent slowly returning my body to a normal 98.6 degrees. Blood was drawn. Computed tomography (CT) scans and X-ray images were taken of my brain and my chest. Tubes were inserted all over my body, into my windpipe and into my nose. Incisions were made to insert more tubes into my veins and arteries, through which heart and pain medication and nutrients would be supplied to my body. Electrodes and wires were attached to measure and monitor my vital signs, in an effort to determine what exactly was happening to my body.

Once they were able to figure out what was going on with my heart, and what was going on with the rest of my body, they would be able to create a plan of action. As they were pouring over all my test results and grainy images of my brain, they were also assessing the damage that had already been done. They were determining the likelihood of any sort of recovery.

I can't imagine how Luke must have felt. Until family started arriving the next morning, Luke was alone. He sat alone in the intensive care waiting room all night, not knowing if his wife, who was still unconscious, was going to live or die. Luke had been scrambling around seemingly non-stop for the past several hours. Luke had administered round after round of CPR, answered hundreds of questions about my medical history, made several difficult phone calls, and cared for his sons in the most chaotic of circumstances. There was nowhere for any of that nervous energy to go, and now there was nothing for him to do but wait.

The arrival of family members didn't do much to break the quiet tension or speed the passage of time. At 4:30 in the morning, Luke's father and the preacher arrived to find Luke on the floor of the waiting room, trying to catch a few minutes of sleep. Luke told them what had happened. He told them that my heart was beating again, but I was unconscious and on life support. The preacher led them in a few prayers in the waiting room. Later, when the sun had come up, family began to appear: my mother; my father and his wife, Laurie; and my sisters, Julie and Susan. This was the first time since our wedding that our families had been together. Everyone spoke quietly and visited nervously with one another while they waited to hear any news.

Early Tuesday morning, a full day after I'd been admitted to the hospital in the very early hours of Monday morning, the doctors called a family conference. Luke was bleary eyed, exhausted from worry and lack of sleep. Luke said that at the time, he thought this was just the beginning of a long night, maybe a long few days. He'd been in the hospital for about 30 hours straight, so far. Luke had tried to sleep on the waiting room floor for just a few minutes at a time, but it hardly made a difference. Luke was still wearing the same clothes he'd thrown on when he left the house late Sunday night.

Luke, eight other family members, and two doctors—my neurologist Dr. Evans and my cardiologist Dr. Martin—crowded into a conference room with no windows. There were three tables pushed together to form a horseshoe shape. A couple of boxes of tissues were on the table closest to the door. Everyone sat down, except for the two doctors. They stood in front of the room as if they were teaching a class. They spoke in the hushed and slow way that people do when they are delivering bad news.

"Carolyn is still in a coma," Dr. Evans began. "The MRI shows very little activity and extensive brain damage, especially in the back of her brain." He went on, saying, "At this point, we can't tell what brain functions have been affected."

The doctors had no idea which parts of my brain functions had been damaged and which parts of my brain had remained intact. They didn't know what brain functions had been impacted as a result of the lack of oxygen to my brain from the cardiac arrest.

After they'd laid out all of the information they knew about my current condition—which wasn't much—they paused. Then, Dr. Evans went on to give my prognosis. That was the information everyone was waiting for. My family wanted to know what my future looked like. Was I going to recover?

"It is not clear whether or not Carolyn will come out of the coma," Doctor Evans said. "Her heart may stop permanently or she could be confined to a long-term care facility for the remainder of her life. She will definitely be blind. At any rate, she will never be the Carolyn you knew. At some point, you will need to consider taking her off life support."

My family was stunned. Some people asked questions, others cried. There were a lot of tears. Overcome with emotion and unable to continue putting on a brave face, Luke quietly walked out of the room, just as the conference ended. In my room in the intensive care unit, Luke stood beside my bed and held my hand. In the ICU, the quiet was punctuated by the high-pitched beeps of the life support machines in the background. The conference room, with its dim lighting and the sound of muffled sobs, had been too quiet. There seemed to be no shadows cast in the bright white fluorescent lighting of my room in the ICU. The disinfectant smell was just as jarring as the bright lights.

Luke says that's when he lost it. He remembers crying and sinking down to the cold white linoleum floor, asking out loud, "Why is this happening? Why is this happening to my Carolyn?" For ten minutes, Luke cried on his knees beside my bed; just clutching my hand and crying, so afraid of losing his wife and the mother of his two young boys, so afraid that this beautiful life that he and his wife had created was over forever.

That morning, questions outnumbered answers. The doctors were uncertain what physical and mental abilities I would retain. No one knew if I would ever be able to walk, talk, or laugh again. Of course, in light of what the doctors had told everyone in the conference room, all of those questions were extremely optimistic. The doctors were uncertain if I would even wake up from the coma, much less talk or walk.

Uncertainty is unsettling, but in uncertainty lies possibility.

Despite the hope provided by the possibility of my waking up and recovering someday, the few certainties established by the doctors were grim. With certainty, the doctors identified areas of severe brain damage to my right and left parietal lobes, the right and left sides of my occipital lobe, and the back of my frontal lobe. Because of this damage, I was going to be blind, according to the doctors. And, according to the doctors, it was certain that I was never going to be the same Carolyn I once was.

I know that my family and friends struggled with all of these uncertainties about my health and recovery. My sisters and my parents in particular were disturbed by Dr. Evans' grim and heavy handed diagnosis. They all started calling him Dr. Doom and Gloom after the conference, and they continue to do so to this day.

But there were other certainties about the situation. These certainties were absent from the doctors' reports and my medical charts; they were certainties that weren't ascertained in CT scans and blood work. I am a fighter, and my family and friends all know that. They know I am stubborn as hell, and they knew I'd do whatever it took to be the best mother to my boys that I possibly could. They knew I would fight to survive.

Ask literally anyone that knows me, and they'll say that I am the most determined and stubborn person they know. I had never before backed down from a challenge, and this wasn't going to be any different. Luke was very much aware of this. He says it's one of the things that gave him strength in those dark days. It's how there in that room in the intensive care unit, where I lay unconscious and attached by so many tubes and wires to life support machines, Luke was able to say to me with confidence that everything was going to be okay. He assured me I was going to make it through all this. His strength gave me strength.

I don't remember Luke's words of encouragement when I was in the ICU, but I know I heard them and I know I sensed his unwavering positivity. It was exactly what I needed. Hearing from Luke, the person for whom my trust knows no bounds, that I was going to get better and that I was still Carolyn, gave me the strength I needed. Even for someone as tough as me though, overcoming such a hopeless prognosis was going to be extremely difficult. I was starting a journey that was going to continue for years.

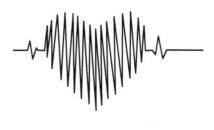

4

Everyone waited.

Each day, the doctors performed a battery of neurological tests on me, watching for signs of life. The EEG and the Head CT scan results showed minimal brain activity. Light pricks on the soles of my feet attempted to elicit some kind of response, a reflexive movement. Nothing. Little flashes of light directly in my eyes, sought a pupil response, some kind of change. No response. No change. My pupils did not shrink in the light. They did not move up, down, or sideways. My eyes were as still as a doll's. Physical therapists bent and stretched my legs, arms, and hands. I didn't move at all.

Friends and family stood vigil by my bedside as I lay unconscious. They held my hands, prayed, and talked to me. Tara, a close friend from high school, massaged my hands with vanilla scented lotion when she came to visit. My sister, Susan, braided my hair. Once I regained consciousness, I looked forward to these little beauty rituals.

Except for waiting, there wasn't much to be done in those first couple weeks that I was in the ICU. My friends and family were all eager for opportunities to help out in any way that they could. Friends brought home cooked meals to the house for Luke and the boys. There were delicious chicken and green bean casseroles, cheesy potatoes, lasagna, and even chocolate cake. One evening, Luke pulled into our driveway after work to find someone mowing our lawn—one of my friends from high school that I hadn't spoken to in years. Family and friends showered Parker and Landon with love and attention and offered to take care of them whenever. I hate that I was not around for my little boys for so long, but they were very well cared for.

When my father and Laurie asked one of the doctors what they could do to help, the doctors told them to buy me some high top sneakers—to keep the tendons in my ankles from shrivelling up and becoming slack. It's something that can happen to someone who is in a lying position and unable to move their legs or ankles for a very extended period of time. If I was ever able to walk again, the high tops would help.

Those high tops were the ugliest shoes I've ever worn. I would've never bought them myself. I do not wear white sneakers. Ever. I am not a basketball player from the 1970s, so I don't wear high tops either. But I wore these.

Visitors started signing their names and writing little messages in colored marker on the white high top canvases. It was one of those little things that helped keep hope alive for everyone. Luke's mom helped Parker and Landon hold the marker in their little hands and write out their names. A lot of the messages said things like,

"We love you Carolyn!"

"We're praying for you!"

"Stay strong!"

Some of my favorites are

"So glad I could hold your hand!"

"Carolyn, I wanna borrow your kicks!"

And of course the message my dad wrote, "Nothing but the best shoes for my Carolyn!"

Those ugly shoes are a treasured keepsake now. They were hideous, but they did what they were supposed to do. When I finally was up on my feet, I was having a lot of problems with balance and muscle weakness, but my ankle tendons were in great shape. My tendons may not have been damaged irreparably, but those shoes helped.

After two days my condition seemed relatively stable. Luke and my family cautiously hoped the worst was over. My heart was still not beating normally. I still experienced dangerous arrhythmias. My heart was beating much too fast. As a result, my heart was not pumping blood through my body efficiently.

Doctors use a measurement called the ejection fraction to describe the heart's efficiency—the percentage of blood that the heart pumps with each beat. Even a healthy heart doesn't pump out all of the blood in the heart with each beat. There's always some blood that remains within the heart, but the less blood that's left in the heart after each beat, the better. My ejection fraction was much too low, meaning that my heart was weak and not pumping blood efficiently. A very low ejection fraction like mine significantly ups the chance of cardiac arrest.

The day after the doctors had given my family the news, it seemed the worst case scenario might really happen: I wouldn't make it out of the hospital. As Luke walked back to the ICU from the restroom, he heard a Code Blue over the PA system. When the announcement gave the room number, Luke said that his heart sank. It was my room number. My heart had stopped again.

When Luke made it to my room just a few minutes later, the doctors had already restarted my heart. It was the second time in three days that my heart had stopped. This time, the doctors were able to quickly restart it, since I was already in the hospital. Defibrillator paddles and prepared injections of medicines to get my heart restarted were at the ready near my bed, but there was no guarantee that this would be the last time I would go into sudden cardiac arrest. And there was no guarantee that if it did stop again, the doctors would be able to restart my heart again. People started to fear that Dr. Evans was right. My heart could stop again, maybe for good. Things didn't look promising.

A week passed. My heart and lung function began to improve. I started to breathe on my own. The doctors and nurses took me off of the ventilator. They left my tracheostomy in, just in case I needed to be put on the ventilator again. My vital signs looked good, but I still didn't show any signs of increased brain activity. The true extent of the brain damage was still unknown.

Somewhere around one hundred fifty people showed up to the hospital to visit and offer their prayers and support. A steady stream of visitors kept the waiting room full. At one point, thirty-five people crowded into the ICU waiting room, waiting to see me. The ICU only allowed visitors in my room in groups of three at a time, during certain hours, and in between frequent tests and examinations.

Luke says the constant presence of visitors helped drown out the constant whine of the machines and monitors. Visitors kept him grounded. When Luke was alone with his thoughts, he'd start to get anxious. The visitors' prayers and kind words to both me and Luke were a welcome break from all the medical jargon. There were a lot of tears. No one really completely broke down, but some were clearly taken aback when they saw me.

Most of my visitors were close friends and family members—friends from work, friends from high school, former teammates from synchronized swimming and field hockey, and friends from college. People that I had lost touch with, people that I had only known passing, and even people I'd never met—friends of friends—came to the hospital to see me.

My junior varsity field hockey coach, Slade, was among these unexpected visitors. I hated her.

Well, I hated her when she was my coach. Slade didn't play me our first game of the season. I was so angry. She knew I was good. She knew I'd been playing for four years longer than any of the other girls on the team, so why couldn't I play? It didn't make any sense, and it wasn't fair.

Naturally, I rolled my eyes and made plenty of sarcastic quips during practice the next week after Slade refused to play me. One warm September afternoon, when Slade thought the team was slacking, Slade made my team run extra sprints. I was tired of running. It had been a long day, and I was not in the best mood. I looked straight at her and crossed my arms. I tilted my head to the left slightly, raised my eyebrows in that way that teenage girls do, and said "I'm not running anymore, and you can't make me."

That did it. The next thing I knew, Slade was up in my face, barking at me. She was not going to let me talk to her like that, and she was not going to let me decide what I was going to do or not do on her field.

"If you don't want to do the extra sprints, you can leave and not come back," Slade told me. Slade didn't mess around.

I did the sprints, but I seethed with anger for the

rest of practice. I somehow managed to tone down the attitude, and we moved on for the most part. But I quietly resented her for the rest of the year.

Years later, while I was pregnant with Parker, Slade and I met again. We both worked at the University of Richmond. I was a dietician, and she was a nurse. When we first ran into each other at a Christmas party at work, I was a little surprised how friendly she was. It was strange talking to Slade as an adult. We were peers now.

"I can't believe you would want to talk to me, after the way I treated you back in high school," I told Slade - half laughing, even though I was serious.

Slade looked me in the eye.

"Carolyn," she said, smiling, "you were in high school. That's how high school girls are. You were growing up and learning a lot of valuable life lessons. I liked that you were headstrong. You were a great player. You reminded me of myself." She smiled again. We were on good terms, and that made me really happy.

The very same personality traits that pitted Slade and I against each other back in my high school days on the field made us friends as adults. We were both strong, out-spoken women. While

Slade and I were friendly, we never got really close, but we did cross paths on occasion. I never saw Slade outside of work. We were both busy and had our own families. We talked about getting our respective departments, the health center and the dining center, to collaborate on programs for students and faculty. But life got in the way, as it does. A few months later, I gave birth to Parker and took maternity leave. We didn't get very far on that project. We both thought there would be plenty of time for that down the road.

When my friend Jaclyn heard that I was in the hospital, she called Slade. Jaclyn also played field hockey with me on Slade's team in high school. Jaclyn wanted more than anything to be there with me in the hospital, but she lived in Boston and couldn't get out to Richmond right away. Jaclyn later told me how she felt helpless so far away. She needed to do something. So she called Slade.

Jaclyn told Slade, "Carolyn is in the hospital and she's dying! You have to do something. You're a nurse!" Jaclyn didn't give Slade details about my condition. Slade didn't know Luke at all, either.

Soon after she received that phone call from Jaclyn, Slade went to the ICU at the hospital in Richmond. She introduced herself to Luke as an old friend of mine. At the time, Slade had no idea what a significant role she would play in my recovery.

Luke and Slade quickly bonded. Since they didn't know each other before, they had a lot to talk about—how they had each met me, where they grew up, what they did for a living, and who were their families. Plus, Slade's husband was a big Red Sox fan, just like Luke. They talked about their lives and each of their memories of me, laughing about the good times.

Luke says talking with her helped take his mind off of what was happening. And that was exactly one of the things that kept him sane. When times were tough, Luke and I supported each other. Now, Luke was going through one of the toughest times of his life, and I wasn't there for him. He very much needed someone strong to give him a little direction and tell him everything was going to turn out okay. Slade ended up being that someone. She was a rock for Luke, and for me as well, even before I knew she was there. She spent time with Luke at my bedside, while I was still unconscious. I don't remember any of this, but I'm told she talked to me just like she used to when she was my coach, saying things like, "You're not going to win just lying there like that Carolyn. You need to just hurry up and wake up!"

Slade watched Luke struggle for about a week to keep track of all the little bits of paper where he was writing things down—appointments, test results, people's schedules, new information about my condition, questions to ask my doctors—before she stepped in and got him organized. Luke kept all the bits of paper crammed in between the pages of a small notebook. Slade could tell that Luke was growing more and more overwhelmed. It seemed like he was always frantically flipping through that notebook.

One day, when Slade was standing by my bed and Luke was sitting in a chair with his little blue spiral notebook, bursting with all those little bits of paper, she looked down at him and said, "How's that organizational system working out for you, buddy?"

At that moment, a couple of pieces of paper fluttered to the ground. Luke laughed and shrugged. Slade went home that night and made Luke a binder with few notebooks to stay organized and keep him sane. The first section of the binder had a calendar for Luke to keep track of when tests were being done, when test results were expected back, when different family members and friends would be at the hospital to visit, and when he was going to go see Parker and Landon. Another section contained a folder for organizing doctor's notes. Slade also left a sizable section for Luke to write down any questions he wanted to ask the doctors. There were always so many questions.

Slade gave Luke a small stack of blank notebooks, too. She told him he should use one as a journal, and she suggested that Luke write down everything he wanted to tell me—stuff about Landon and Parker, what was happening at work, things he wanted to tell me once I was better, and any other thoughts that were weighing on him. Luke was grateful. Slade said after she gave him the binder and the notebooks, he looked a little less lost.

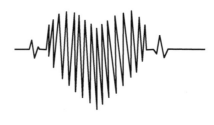

5

Not long after I'd been admitted to the hospital, one of my friends created a Facebook page, titled "Get Well Carolyn!" to keep my family and friends informed about my progress. On July 17th, the day that Luke and I had planned on leaving for our vacation to Florida, Luke made the following post to my Facebook page:

> *Just letting everyone know that in my eyes Carolyn made an attempt to tell me she was thirsty today. She can't speak right now with the trache in but her tongue pressed against her teeth and her lips moved and appeared to say thirsty. The doctor said not to get my hopes up, but I have been in that room every day and never saw anything close to that thus far.*

Regaining consciousness was a gradual process for me. I didn't snap out of the coma like people do in soap operas. I didn't suddenly open my eyes, sit straight up, and start asking questions. When I did start to gain consciousness, I didn't want to know where I was, what day it was, and what had happened. For two weeks, I was in a kind of liminal state not entirely conscious but not unconscious, and it was months before I could sit up on my own.

At first, my eyelids started to flutter. A few days later, I started opening my eyes and blinking slowly for a few minutes. Gradually, my eyes stayed open for longer periods of time. Even when my eyes were open, it was hard to tell if I was still there. My gaze was totally unfocused. I've been told I looked like a doll, lying there with glassy, faraway eyes. Where was I? I can't remember anything from that time, so I can't say. I can say I wasn't entirely lost. I had so many people that loved me there at my side to help me find my way back.

To my family, just seeing my eyes opening and closing seemed to be a good sign, but the doctors cautioned them against getting too excited. They still didn't know what level of brain function I would retain. At this point, it was still a definite possibility that I would either remain in a vegetative state or have very limited mental capacity. Dr. Doom and Gloom made sure to emphasize that. It's common for people in vegetative states to open their eyes. The doctors still thought there was no way I would be the same Carolyn. So the waiting continued.

A few days after I started opening my eyes, I started trying to talk. I was breathing on my own and off the ventilator, but I still had a tracheostomy tube in my throat. I couldn't talk with the tracheostomy tube in, but Luke could see I was trying. The first time he saw me trying to talk, he said it looked like I was trying to say that I was thirsty. My tongue pressed up against my teeth, and my lips moved in such a way that it looked like I was trying to say the word "thirsty." Luke texted Slade to tell her the good news. She advised Luke to place his finger over my trache for a few seconds so I could make sounds. He did. My voice was soft and garbled sounding, but Luke could just make out "I'm thirsty," and "I love you."

With these attempts, Luke could see the frustration in my eyes that I wasn't able to properly express myself. A couple days later, Luke called my father and told him, "Someone wants to talk to you." Luke nodded to the nurse, and she placed her finger over the hole in the trache. He held the receiver close to my mouth, and I mumbled a few words into the phone. My voice sounded raspy. It was impossible for Luke or my father on the other end of the phone to translate my garbled sounding words, but that was all beside the point. It didn't matter what I was trying to say; I was talking. I was alive. I wasn't a vegetable. I was talking. Luke could hear the joy in my father's voice on the other end of the line.

My incoherent mumblings quickly became words. Soon, I was stringing the words into sentences. Over the course of 24 hours, I'd gone from making throaty noises to asking questions and stating my opinion on the temperature of the room. Luke clearly remembers the day a nurse asked him to leave my room, because I was talking too much and needed to rest.

"Is it too early to talk?"

"When can I eat?"

"It is so hot!"

"What is the deal?"

These were some of the things I said that stuck out in Luke's mind.

My speech was still far from perfect though. When Luke had told Dr. Evans what I was saying, he shrugged it off. It's common for people in a vegetative state to speak in short sentences, he said. Dr. Evans said I probably didn't know what I was saying. Some of what I said was a little random and nonsensical, but some of it wasn't.

Despite Dr. Evans' pessimism, Luke was confident that I was still there. Luke could tell I was frustrated that I couldn't communicate very well. There were subtle signs of frustration—little sighs, changes in my tone of voice. But to Luke, the fact that I was frustrated meant that I was feeling emotion and that I knew what I was saying. It meant awareness. As hard as it was for him to know I was upset, he knew it was a good sign.

To prevent my heart from stopping again, the doctors implanted a device in my heart that functions as both a pacemaker and a defibrillator. This device, called an implantable cardioverter defibrillator (ICD), would detect any arrhythmia and immediately correct it by administering electrical pulses to restore a normal heart rhythm. Once my heart and lung function improved, a surgeon implanted the ICD. This surgery took place on July 24th.

This was the same device that I'd asked about having implanted when I was first diagnosed. Implanting this kind of device does have associated risks. Infection, perforation of the heart, and internal bleeding are all possible complications. At the time I was diagnosed, my Long QT Syndrome was not considered severe enough to warrant the risks associated with having an ICD implanted. My situation was very different after the cardiac arrest. I was no longer the strong and healthy, athletic woman with only the slightest risk that LQTS would pose any problems for me. I was now a survivor of sudden cardiac arrest.

The surgery went well, and there were no complications.

Once the ICD was implanted and my condition was clearly stable, plans were made for me to be discharged from the ICU. On July 28th, I left the hospital in Richmond to continue my recovery at a rehabilitation hospital at the University of Virginia in Charlottesville. The rehabilitation hospital at UVA had the facilities and the medical specialist professionals that I needed to help me overcome severe problems with my vision, mobility, memory, and motor skills. These specialists were going to help me get back to being a mommy.

Selecting a rehabilitation hospital hadn't been easy. Originally, we planned on me going to a great rehabilitation hospital in Richmond, at the Medical College of Virginia, MCV. Luke could still see the boys every night, since it was close to our home, and it was one of the best rehabilitation hospitals in the country. After Luke filed all the necessary paperwork and my medical records were sent over, MCV replied that I wasn't healthy enough for their program yet. The next day, we got word that our second choice, the rehabilitation hospital at UVA, had accepted me, but we had to decide if we would take the bed within 24 hours. UVA only had a limited number of beds available. Like the rehabilitation hospital at MCV, the rehabilitation hospital at UVA was one of the best in the country, but it was 80 miles away from our home.

Luke was faced with a difficult choice. We could wait a few weeks to see if my health improved enough for MCV to accept me into their program, or I could go to UVA now. Time was of the essence. All of my doctors had emphasized how important early rehabilitation is for people who have sustained severe brain injuries. The first month is critical, and we were approaching the one-month mark fast. As difficult as it would be to have me so far from home, Luke decided getting me into UVA right away would be best.

Before I even arrived, UVA assigned three therapists to work with me: Theresa for physical therapy, Mallory for speech therapy, and Erica for occupational therapy. I distinctly recall the ambulance ride from the ICU to UVA, but I don't remember meeting my therapists.

I don't actually have any memory of the three weeks I spent in the ICU at the hospital in Richmond. Everything I know of that time, Luke, family, and friends pieced together from their memories. I started to show signs of regaining consciousness after about a week and a half from the time I was admitted to the ICU, late at night on July 5th. In those first few weeks of regaining consciousness, my short-term memory did not function well. I could hold my own in simple conversations, but I couldn't really remember what I had done or said five minutes later.

On the one hand, I hate that there's over an entire month that I just don't remember. I'm a type A personality, and I like to know what's going on so I can feel like I have some control in a situation. I'm someone who likes to have my say. On the other hand, I think regaining awareness slowly made it easier to accept what had happened to me. I think slowly realizing the extent of the damage in my brain was less traumatic than if I would've had the mental capacity to take all this in right away. It almost seemed like a self-preservation mechanism: there was so much for me to mentally and emotionally process, but I wasn't capable of processing very much for a few weeks, so it was a naturally gradual process.

I do remember the trip in the ambulance from the hospital in Richmond to the rehab hospital in Charlottesville. While I remember the ambulance ride, I don't remember arriving at the hospital. I don't remember taking the elevator to the second floor where my room was. I don't remember meeting any of my therapists. The memories I do have of the first few days at the rehab hospital are few and scattered. Those six weeks are gone to me. Except for that ambulance ride, almost an entire month exists between one memory and the next.

I think the memory of the ambulance ride sticks out because I was in so much pain. I remember laying on my back on a stretcher in the ambulance and crying out in pain, "Help me! Help me! My body, it hurts!"

The pain was indescribable. Without a doubt, it was a ten on the UPAT. On the Universal Pain Assessment Tool, that chart that you might have seen in a hospital or doctor's office that shows a 0 to 10 scale, with corresponding drawings of faces for each interval, each face looks increasingly distraught. A ten on the scale is "Worst

Possible Pain." On this scale, zero is no pain, a six is considered Moderate Pain that "interferes with tasks and concentration," and an eight, Severe Pain, "interferes with basic needs."

This pain eclipsed everything. My entire body hurt. Every single one of the muscles in my body was throbbing in pain. The pain felt similar to a charley horse, but worse, so much worse, and all over my entire body. Imagine a persistent charley horse happening to all of the muscles in your body at once that doesn't go away.

Why was I experiencing such agonizing pain? At the time, I wasn't asking myself this question. I was in so much pain that I couldn't think about anything else besides being in pain. I didn't care why it was happening. I just wanted it to stop. After the pain medication took effect and the pain subsided a bit, I did start to wonder what was causing it. Later, I learned that the pain I experienced was caused by muscle spasms, or spasticity— an extreme stiffening of the muscles. It's caused by damage to nerve pathways in the brain that control muscle movement. This was yet another way that the lack of oxygen had damaged my brain.

Unfortunately, this wasn't an isolated incident. The pain in my muscles was constant, and it was worse at night. I would wake up in the middle of the night crying because my muscles hurt so badly. Instantly, Luke appeared at my side, massaging my muscles and softly reassuring me in the dark that we'd get some pain medicine for me, and it would start working very soon. Luke buzzed the nurse's station, and they came in to give me more pain medicine. The pain medicine was strong, but it always seemed to wear off well before I could have another dose.

The muscle pain remained unbearable for a week. After the first week at the rehab hospital, the spastic pain gradually subsided, but the muscle stiffness remained. Although the pain subsided, I was still unable to move the way I used to. I couldn't pick things up. I couldn't sit upright, I couldn't stand up, and I certainly couldn't walk. For months, my legs, arms, and shoulders twitched involuntarily. The twitching was sometimes violent and was especially bad in my shoulders. I probably looked like a robot, short-circuiting.

Trying to make my body do anything was like trying to play a song on a very out of tune piano or a piano that's been pushed out of a seventh story window. Not only is the piano out of tune, but the notes are just wrong, and the wrongness is random.

When I spoke, sometimes I would say the wrong word, even though I knew the right word in my head. If I tried to extend my right arm straight in front of me, something entirely different happened, like my right arm bent at the elbow instead of extending straight in front of me. I guess that's what the doctors meant when they said that I was not capable of any purposeful movements.

I felt so broken, yet my body was mostly intact. Besides my brain, my body had sustained no physical damage. The rigid muscle pain eventually subsided. However, the damage to my brain was significant. The wiring was damaged. The electrical system in my heart had short-circuited and caused my heart to stop working. Now, the short-circuiting of the neurons in the damaged parts of my brain were making it difficult to move, to see, and to speak.

Even my heart itself had incurred little structural damage. A sudden cardiac arrest is completely different from a heart attack. People often think the two are one in the same, but they are very different. In a heart attack, the flow of blood to the heart is blocked, but the heart actually keeps beating. After a heart attack, the heart muscle is damaged. In effect, a portion of the heart muscle actually dies from lack of oxygen. Blood carries oxygen, and if the blood supply is cut off to part of the heart, it doesn't receive oxygen. The extent of the damage can vary, but there is always a certain degree of damage to the heart muscle. In a sudden cardiac arrest, the heart muscle itself is usually okay. My heart muscle was a little weaker. But now that my heart's normal rhythm was restored and I was outfitted with an ICD, my heart was in pretty good shape—much better shape than my brain.

Looking at the head CT scans, the doctors saw that the damage was widespread throughout my brain. My right and left parietal lobes, the right and left sides of my occipital lobe, and the back of my frontal lobe were all damaged. All of these parts of the brain are watershed areas. The watershed areas of the brain are the most vulnerable to damage when the brain is deprived of oxygen. It is the watershed areas that are usually the first areas in the brain where neurons start dying when the brain is deprived of oxygen, such as in the event of cardiac arrest or a stroke.

Each of these parts of the brain has a number of associated functions, so it's difficult to predict what kinds of lasting effects will result from a brain injury based on a CT scan. Blindness, any number of

mobility problems, severe memory problems, diffi-
culty writing and speaking, emotional problems,
and impaired reasoning skills, to name a few were
all likely outcomes of the injuries I had sustained to
these watershed areas of the brain.

What abilities would I lose forever? What
abilities would I be able to regain? Only time would
tell how the damage to the wiring in my brain
would manifest itself.

Luke has always been an amazing father and
husband. He's as much a super dad as I'm a super
mom. If he hadn't already qualified for father and
husband of the year before, he certainly did now.
He didn't have to stay with me every night at the
rehab hospital, but he did. Driving the eighty miles
from Richmond to Charlottesville every day wasn't
feasible, but Luke wanted to be there with me every
day.

Luke slept in a chair those first few nights at
UVA. He was perfectly willing to do this for the next
few months, but the hospital let Luke sleep in the
empty bed in my room. While Luke tirelessly cared
for me, he continued to go to work and regularly
visit the boys, who stayed in Ashland with Luke's
parents.

The doctors at UVA continued to administer neurological tests on me. The tests that they administered became increasingly sophisticated. By the time I left the ICU, I was able to pass the tests that assessed the most basic brain functioning. However, I was having a hard time with some of the tests therapists did when I first arrived at UVA.

"If it's 1:00 now, what time will it be in one hour?" a nurse asked.

I had no idea. I started crying. I knew it was something I should know, but I didn't know how to or couldn't find the answer in my brain. I couldn't even venture a guess.

"It's okay," she reassured me. "It'll come. It'll all come back. You just have to practice."

Sometimes the nurse or the therapist asked me to spell words. A nurse asked me to spell "world" both forwards and backwards. I could spell it forwards, but not backwards. Things like this happened a lot in the beginning. The connections in my brain seemed scrambled. I wanted to say one thing, but I actually said another. I tried to move my arm one way, and it either moved another way or didn't move at all. All of the information I needed to function seemed to be still in my brain, but I wasn't able to access the information the way I used to. It was frustrating and bewildering not being able to always express myself accurately.

Besides mixing up words and having trouble finding the right words, I didn't have much trouble with my speech. Apparently the damage to that part of my brain was very limited. So instead of working on my speech in speech therapy, the therapist and I first started working on my memory. After my brain had more time to heal, we began working on writing and reading

The first session of speech therapy was very emotionally difficult. My speech therapist, Mallory, asked questions to me designed to assess my memory.

"What is Parker's middle name?" she asked.

"Who is the president of the United States?"

"What is Luke's phone number?"

I had no idea. If Mallory prompted me with the first letter, I could sometimes remember. When she hinted that Parker's middle name starts with a W, I remembered. Wade. Once I recalled something, it stuck. It was the initial accessing of memories that was difficult.

I didn't have trouble talking, but because I was on so much medication, the things I said could be quite strange. This made for many amusing conversations. I talked about cabana boys with Luke.

When my friend, Tara, came to visit me, apparently I thought she was wearing black lace lingerie. I kept asking her why she was wearing lingerie in public and mentioned to other friends, "Tara was totally wearing lingerie when she came to see me. Black, lace lingerie. What is up with that?"

After a couple of weeks, when I was finally off most of the drugs and was clear-headed again, I was ready to see what was inside of this body. I was ready to prove the doctors wrong. I had already proven much of their prognosis wrong. I came out of the coma. I wasn't a vegetable. I could talk. My vision was bad, but I wasn't totally blind. And I was still the same Carolyn, the same feisty, stubborn, Carolyn who would do anything for her two sons. I won't be able to walk again? Just watch me!

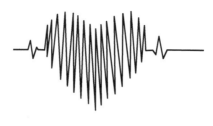

6

Early in my second week in the ICU in Richmond, when the extent of the brain damage was still unknown, my sister Susan swears that I tried to tell her to take out my tubes. She distinctly remembers me mouthing the words, "Take it out. It hurts."

Tubes were coming out of virtually every hole in my body. Tubes in my throat, in my nose, in my stomach, in my arms, in my chest, tubes everywhere. When Susan told the doctors about my early attempts to talk, they summarily dismissed her. Dr. Evans kept reminding my family that the brain scans and neurological tests indicated only very limited brain activity. Based on these tests, there was just no way I'd be talking. My requests went unfulfilled.

Of course, even if they had believed Susan, the

doctors and nurses wouldn't have taken out any of the tubes. Whether I found them to be uncomfortable or not was not the issue; the tubes were connected to the very machines keeping me alive in the ICU.

When I arrived at the rehab hospital at UVA, I was off of life support. The only tubes still connected to my body were the catheter and the feeding tube. My recovery in the hospital was marked by the removal of each of these tubes.

Each removal of each tube was an important milestone. Luke and I both remember the dates each one of them were removed: the ventilator tube came out on July 17th; the tracheostomy tube was removed a week later, on July 23rd; the catheter tube was removed on August 7th; and the feeding tube—the last tube—was removed on August 31st.

Every time the doctors removed a tube, it meant that my health was improving. My body began regaining strength and the ability to perform its essential functions on its own, without the help of machines. It meant the end of a lot of discomfort. And it meant independence. In my mind, the removal of each tube brought me one step closer to getting back to being a mommy to Landon and Parker.

My catheter was removed for good on August 7th, about a week and a half after I arrived at the rehab hospital. I was happy to have the catheter out and not have to deal with painful urinary tract infections and the constant general discomfort anymore.

While the discomforts of having a catheter were over, I now faced a new set of challenges: getting to the toilet. When the nurses removed my catheter, my weakened body was still a long way from walking. Not being able to even sit up by myself at this point, an entire team of nurses had to assist me every time I needed to pee. It was such a production when the nurses were involved, and I felt more comfortable with Luke. Luke helped me use the toilet in the morning.

Any other time I needed to use the toilet, a nurse positioned a portable toilet next to my bed. Two nurses lifted me up out of the bed or out of the wheelchair and a third nurse pulled down my pants and helped me wipe. It was embarrassing every time.

The constipation from all the pain medication was a welcome side effect. One less thing to deal with. There were times when I almost missed having a catheter and not having to deal with all the embarrassment and the hassle. While Luke was at work during the day, I tried to hold it as long as possible. The nurses helped me to the toilet before lunch, and then I could usually wait until Luke got back to the hospital from work in the evening. Despite these challenges, I knew getting the catheter out was a step in moving forward and recovering.

The staff and the facilities at the rehab hospital were great, but it was hard to get a good night's sleep there. Most days, a nurse came into my room to take blood at 5:00 in the morning, before the sun even came up. Even if I hadn't fallen asleep until 4:00 a.m. and was completely exhausted, I could never fall back to sleep after the nurse came to take blood. There's something about being jabbed with needles . . .

On top of waking up far too early because of nurses doing blood work on me, I constantly woke up during the night because of various noises. Every night, for example, housekeeping came into my room to empty the trash somewhere between the hours of midnight and 3:00 a.m. They always made sure it was well after both Luke and I had fallen asleep. It doesn't seem like something like that would have to be a particularly disruptive operation, but it was. I could distinctly make out the sound of each part of the procedure: fumbling around with the garbage can to get the bag out, shaking open the new bag, and stuffing it in the garbage can.

I had a friend who had a dog that would pee on the floor every time he heard someone shaking open a garbage bag because it scared him so much. I'm not saying these noises scared me so much I peed, but they were just the kind of sound I couldn't sleep through.

Maybe the combination of being sleep deprived and in constant pain caused me to be a little more sensitive to the disruptions in my sleep, but I had a tendency to not let the fact that I had been woken up go unnoticed. Usually I would just glare at the offender and say "Are you serious? Are you seriously doing this right now?"

One night, a confused nurse's assistant stumbled into the wrong room and woke me up to change my diaper. "Are you wet?" he asked, lightly shaking me awake.

I was not having it. "Am I wet? I don't even wear a freaking diaper!" My language may or may not have been more colorful than what I've written here.

Every morning, Luke woke up early and got himself ready for the day. He kept his tooth brush, tooth paste, shaving cream, and razor in a little travel caddy. Luke traveled often for work. Ever the optimist, he'd just say he was used to living out of suitcases.

Once Luke showered and dressed for the day, he helped me get ready for the day. He was so gentle and so thorough in everything he did for me. At times, I felt like a burden, not being able to do anything for myself, but it certainly was not because of anything Luke said or did. I couldn't help thinking that surely Luke had no idea this was in store for him when we were married and he vowed to have and to hold me, from that day forward…in sickness and in health. But Luke took it all in stride. He was all smiles, like always. Luke was so loving and happy when he was with me that I didn't tend to be bothered by those thoughts for long.

Luke started the day off by helping me to the toilet. Next, he gave me a sponge bath. (Let me tell you, a sponge bath is a lousy substitute for a hot shower, but it was better than nothing.) After the sponge bath, Luke brushed my teeth and then styled my long, curly, dark brown hair.

Notice I didn't say brush. You can't brush hair that's as curly as mine. As soon as you run a brush through it, it turns into a big pouf ball, like one of those awful hair styles from the 1980s. To make my hair look good, Luke had to wet it, add a dollop of mouse, and scrunch it—the same way I had to when I could style my own hair. A lot of the nurses would try to brush it. That's why my sister, Susan, braided it in those first few weeks in the ICU—to keep anyone from brushing it.

There was one nurse at UVA whose daughter had curly hair. That nurse knew better. I even offered her some tips on techniques for how to best style her daughter's curly hair. The daughter was very grateful. The nurse told me how excited her daughter was when a few of the tips I told her about worked well for her daughter's own hair. The nurse's daughter was 12, that age when girls start caring a little bit more about what they look like.

It took some effort to teach Luke how to style my hair properly, especially since I couldn't show him what to do. Teaching my husband how to properly style long curly hair through verbal instruction alone was a challenge. Luke's a fast learner though, and within a week, he made a fabulous beautician for my hair.

The sudden role reversal struck me, especially when Luke dressed me in the mornings, guiding my arms through the sleeves of my t-shirt, pulling the shirt gently over my head, just like a parent dressing a baby does. A month ago, I had been doing all of these things for my baby boys. I bathed them, dressed them, and fed them. Now, I couldn't do any of these things for myself. If I couldn't take care of myself, how was I going to manage to take care of two babies?

Thinking of this, I felt defeated sometimes. It could be hard not to feel this way. When I started to lose hope, I tried to remind myself that I was still here, alive against all odds. I was alive; alive to love my boys, alive to watch my children grow.

Being able to be present for my children was huge, but I didn't want to just be present. I wanted to raise my children with my husband. I needed to get better for Landon and Parker, and feeling sorry for myself wasn't going to get me up and moving any faster. I didn't have children so that someone else could raise them. This motivation planted itself in the forefront of my mind early on in my recovery. It's what got me through the tough days.

The feeding tube came out last, on August 31st. It stuck out of my midsection, an inch to the left of my bellybutton. The tube was attached to the inside wall of my stomach. Swallowing was one of the many functions that my brain couldn't remember how to carry out. Trouble swallowing, which is called dysphagia, is common in people who suffer brain damage due to a lack of oxygen to the brain. The doctors hoped this would be only a temporary issue, and it was. Aspirating food or liquids into the lungs is always a serious concern for people with dysphagia. Choking is an obvious danger and so is pneumonia. A severe infection like pneumonia was absolutely the last thing my body needed. I wouldn't be able to eat until I successfully completed a swallow study in order to confirm that I was able to swallow.

Three times a day, a nurse brought a can of formula into my room and poured it into my feeding tube—more like taking medicine than eating a meal. I didn't feel hungry, but eventually, not being able to eat got pretty old.

While I was still on the feeding tube, my dietician decided to try a bulk feeding. This involved administering a day's worth of formula all at once. One feeding a day was more convenient for the nurses than three. It was the first and last time we tried it! Not even 20 minutes after my "meal," I had a case of dumping syndrome, which is exactly what it sounds like. One of my friends was in my room, visiting, at the time. She paged the nurse to help me to the toilet, but the nurse didn't arrive in time. Fortunately, my friend bravely stepped in and helped me to the toilet herself. To this day, whenever I remember that afternoon, I feel both grateful and mortified.

After weeks of not being able to eat or drink anything by mouth, I found myself longing for an ice cold Sprite® and a slice of pizza from my favorite pizza place in Charlottesville—Mellow Mushroom®. When I was doing my dietetic internship in Charlottesville, the other interns and I always went out for pizza at Mellow Mushroom® on Fridays. My cravings for Sprite® and pizza were more intense than the cravings I had for shrimp when I was pregnant with Landon and Parker, and those were intense!

Seeing and smelling the trays of hospital food that Luke ate for dinner didn't bother me. It was hospital food (i.e. it hardly resembled real food). But seeing non-hospital food was hard. I remember one afternoon when Luke's parents—Dee-Dee and Pop-Pop to the boys—stopped by with the boys after they'd gone apple picking at Carter's Mountain. Landon was eating some of Carter's legendary home-made apple cider donuts. What I would've done for a bite of that soft, sugary goodness! The swallow test couldn't come fast enough.

Seeing and smelling those donuts—real, delicious food—was hard, but having a feeding tube made things easier for me in a way. With a feeding tube, I didn't have to feed myself, or perhaps more accurately, I didn't have to be fed by someone else. For several weeks, I couldn't hold a spoon or a fork to feed myself. Using a knife to cut my food was completely out of the question. When I was able to hold a fork in my hand, I couldn't see the food on my plate. Even if I could hold my fork and see my food, I couldn't have successfully maneuvered the fork to bring the food to my mouth. My brain had to relearn to use these muscles all over again.

As much as I missed eating and as much as having a feeding tube was uncomfortable, this tube allowed me to not think about just one of the many simple things I couldn't do anymore. It was the same with the catheter. I hated having it in, but having it out meant I had to confront a new set of challenges. I knew I was going to be able to feed myself eventually, but I also knew it was going to be a long and difficult road.

When I was studying to be a dietician, I learned all about feeding tubes. I spent four years and an internship learning about them. When I worked at a long-term care facility after my internship, a big part of my job was to prescribe formula for patients with feeding tubes. It was my first job out of school. I thought I knew everything there was to know about feeding tubes. I thought I knew all about the precautions that needed to be taken.

What I didn't learn from the textbooks and the lectures was what it would actually feel like to have a feeding tube. I didn't understand what an accidental pull or snag on a patient's feeding tube felt like. Nurses and even friends visiting did it all the time on accident, and each time I'd yowl in pain. A sharp pain, like someone poking around in an open wound, flared at the site of the tube. In school, we learned that bulk feedings could cause digestive distress in some patients but wouldn't have any lasting effects on their health. We didn't learn what the digestive distress was really like. We didn't have a clue what the pain or the ensuing embarrassment actually felt like. It's just not something someone can learn from textbooks and lectures.

The weight loss started while I had the feeding tube in. I don't think they were giving me enough calories. I've always been thin. Before I was admitted to the hospital, I weighed 123 pounds. For my height, 5 foot 8 inches, that's considered a healthy weight, but on the thinner end of the spectrum. While I was in the hospital, I lost just over 10 pounds. That might not seem like a great deal of weight to lose, but I didn't have much to lose to begin with. I was significantly underweight. I looked frail. I lost muscle as well. The contours and shapes of each of my bones became visible under my skin. Running my hands along my body, I could feel each individual rib of my ribcage. Once the feeding tube was out and I started eating again, I continued to lose weight. Relearning how to walk, take care of myself, and take care of my kids while getting back to a healthy weight was going to be a challenge.

One wouldn't think I used up that much energy laying in a hospital bed and sitting in a wheelchair most of the day. I had regular physical therapy, but the therapists weren't exactly having me run laps or do bench presses. Nevertheless, my brain and my muscles no longer knew the most efficient way to use energy and complete movements, so each movement I made required much more energy than it did before my brain was damaged.

I used an incredible amount of energy to complete even the smallest and most ordinary movements and tasks. My brain and my muscles needed to relearn everything. When I did sit-ups in physical therapy, I used all my muscles except my stomach muscles. I made a conscious effort to use only my stomach muscles, but it was no use. Even showering while sitting down was tiring. After a month of sponge baths, a nurse helped me shower once a week. I couldn't squeeze the body wash into my palm for a long time, so the nurse did it for me. I knew where my arms and legs were, but I had trouble making my hands move where I wanted them to move. I could see my hands flailing around, moving vaguely in the direction I wanted them to go, but not quite getting to their destination. I was always fumbling.

Regardless, I was determined to get control of my swallows.

The swallow study was the only thing standing between me and a slice of Mellow Mushroom® pizza. By the time August 5th finally rolled around, I was more than a little excited to be able to eat and drink again. An ambulance took me to the radiology department at the main UVA hospital campus. As I sat in my wheelchair, a technician positioned an x-ray machine near me. He explained to me that the x-ray machine would broadcast a live video of my esophagus as I swallowed liquids and solids onto a monitor for the radiologist to observe. I first had to drink a small glass of liquid chalk. If I was able to drink this first drink without any problems, I would progress to the next step, which involved eating some crackers accompanied by a thinner—but still chalky tasting—liquid. The technician held the Styrofoam cup of the thick chalky liquids up to my lips for me to sip and fed me the wafer-thin crackers. The chalky cocktails and the crackers all went down with no problem. Swallow study passed!

Even though I still had the actual tube in my stomach, my doctors gave me the go-ahead to start eating and drinking as soon as I passed the swallow study. That evening, Luke picked up a cheese and mushroom pizza and a cold Sprite® from Mellow Mushroom®. I didn't know pizza could taste so good. For the remainder of my stay at the rehab hospital, Luke brought take-out food back to the hospital from almost every restaurant in Charlottesville.

I passed the swallow study just in time for Luke's and my five-year wedding anniversary. Luke and I enjoyed our anniversary dinner in the hospital room. He brought dinner in from my favorite seafood restaurant in town, Bonefish Bar and Grill.

We went there every year for our anniversary. We feasted on Bang Bang Shrimp and crab cakes with creamy red remoulade sauce, reminiscing about the past five years. The shrimp, lightly breaded, was crispy and had just the right amount of spice. The crab cakes were sweet and fresh with a salty hint of dill. Everything tasted better than I remembered.

Luke and I had shared so many beautiful moments, and we'd been through so much. We talked about how and where we first met. Luke and I were both waiting tables at a seafood restaurant in Nags Head. I was nineteen; Luke was twenty-three. We talked and joked around while we were working, but we didn't start dating until the end of the summer. For our first date, we watched a romantic comedy at Luke's place on the couch. It doesn't sound like the most amazing date ever, but it was magic. After the movie we talked all night about everything. From then on, we were inseparable.

There wasn't a moment when I thought "He's the one," because I think I knew it all along. I could tell he genuinely cared about me. Luke wasn't thinking, "What's in it for me?"

Three years later, we got married. The only reasons Luke and I waited three years to get married were because we were both young and we both wanted to finish school first. Had we been older, we probably would've been married within a year of our first date. And here we were . . . together through the sickness, five years later.

My feeding tube wasn't taken out until August 31st, three weeks later. Apparently scheduling the removal of the feeding tube was an issue, which seemed especially strange after it finally happened. A nurse literally just yanked it out, and after two (very painful) attempts, the tube was out. All in all, it was over in about 30 seconds.

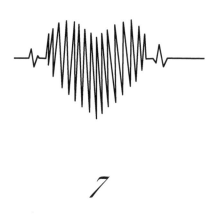

7

I don't know what I would've done without Luke and all my friends and family that came to spend time with me. In the first few months of my stay at UVA, I spent a good part of my day in therapy, but I still spent a lot of time in my room. Luke always made sure that someone came to my room to sit and talk with me every day, but a pretty steady stream of visitors dropped in, as well. My mother was a teacher and had the summer off, so she came by most days to sit and talk with me. Luke's uncle and Slade frequently visited, too.

I appreciated seeing everyone who came to visit me and help me while away the long hours, but I looked most forward to seeing my two favorite visitors: Landon and Parker. The boys stopped to visit over lunchtime, usually once a week with Dee-Dee and Pop-Pop.

When Debbie and Mike brought the boys to my room, Landon always made sure that he was the first one off the elevator. After only a few visits, he knew exactly how to get to my room from the elevator. As soon as the elevator doors opened just enough for his little two-year-old body to fit through, Landon took off through the receding doors. Landon jumped out from the elevator and peered down the hallway to make sure he was about to set off in the right direction. He looked left, then right, and then took off running towards my room in that adorable way that toddlers run, shouting "Mommy! Mommy!"

Landon was (and still is) my wild child. I wish I could've let him jump into my lap! Every time Landon came racing into my room, grinning and declaring himself, yelling "Mommy I'm here!" my heart soared.

"Hey buddy! I missed you so much!" I'd tell him.

I wanted so much to be able to scoop him up and hug him and kiss his soft cheeks! That would have to wait, but I knew it would happen. Instead, all I could do was tell him I was happy to see him and that I loved him.

After he finished his lunch, Landon played on the floor by my bed. We kept a supply of puzzles, books, and toys in my room for Landon and Parker's visits. I couldn't sit on the floor and play with Landon like I used to, so I watched him and talked to him from my wheelchair. It briefly crossed my mind that reading to Landon might be a good substitute to playing with him on the floor like I used to. Unfortunately, my poor vision made this absolutely impossible. I couldn't see well enough to read at all. I wouldn't have been able to turn the pages either. I didn't have the coordination yet.

I used to read to Landon every night when I tucked him into bed. Most nights, I read him his favorite, *I Love You Forever*, by Robert Munsch. The story begins with a mother rocking her new baby to sleep. As her baby grows, she continues to rock him, "back and forth, back and forth." Even when he is a grown man, the mother sometimes sneaks in his house at night and rocks him in his sleep. I didn't know when I'd be able to read again, but I still remembered the words to the song in Munsch's book that the mother sings when she rocks her son: "I'll love you forever, I'll like you for always, as long as I'm living, my baby you'll be."

I missed holding Landon, but not being able to hold Parker was especially hard for me. He was so small during the first month when I was at the rehab hospital. Parker stayed in the baby carrier. He sat right by me, but I could barely see him. I wanted to snuggle him so bad. My arms ached to hold him. As I started to slowly gain more control of my muscles, Debbie would sit Parker on my lap, wrapping my arms around him in an embrace. It wasn't quite the same, but I could still smell his sweet baby smell and feel his warm little body against mine. If I bent my head down, I could feel his impossibly soft skin against my cheek. That intoxicating sweet baby smell doesn't last long. I felt frustrated that I was missing out on a lot of snuggling with my baby. The frustration I felt wasn't all bad though. It fueled my determination to keep working hard in therapy so I could get back to taking care of Landon and Parker as soon as possible.

Debbie stood close by, within arm's reach, when Parker sat on my lap. Of course I wanted her to be there. I was grateful that she was there. It was possible that, through no fault of my own, Parker could roll off my lap. My arms—still weak, stiff, and uncoordinated–could not catch him if he started to squirm and roll away. But I couldn't help wondering, would someone always need to be there? How long would it be until I was well enough to take care of my own sons myself?

Seeing Parker and Landon always renewed my determination to keep working hard in therapy.

Landon was obviously pumped to see me when he came to visit, but he quickly adjusted to not seeing me every day. I think it would've been harder for me if Landon would've had a hard time adjusting to his new schedule. Landon and Parker stayed with their Dee-Dee and Pop-Pop while I worked through therapy, so they were always close to family. Dee-Dee and Pop-Pop took good care of both Landon and Parker. I am so grateful for all of their help.

Dee-Dee and Pop-Pop took the boys on frequent, fun outings—like to the library for story time (but Landon was more interested in the train tables in the children's section), the playground, and even to the river house. At two-years old, I don't think Landon really understood what was going on. Parker definitely didn't.

When I was admitted to the hospital, Parker was only two months old. In a way, I'm glad Landon and Parker were so young when this happened. They likely wouldn't remember. At such a young age, kids tend to be adaptable. Not all kids are, but mine fortunately were. Had this happened when they were older and in school, I think it would've disrupted their lives more. They would've understood what was going on, and it no doubt would've been upsetting.

When Luke got back from work in the evenings, he took me for walks, pushing me in my wheelchair around the hospital grounds. Charlottesville is known for its fall colors. My stay at the rehab hospital went from August to November, so I was there for peak season, when the fall colors were at their brightest. The rehab hospital where I stayed was actually located on the outskirts of Charlottesville in a wooded area. There were even more trees here than there were in the city. Every shade of red, orange, and gold imaginable showed their colors on the tree leaves. I only knew what the fall colors looked like because I'd seen them before, when I did my dietetic internship in Charlottesville. My bad vision made it difficult to even see colors. They were muted, blurred—not very bright at all.

But I enjoyed the fall in my own way. To me, looking at the trees was a little like looking at an impressionist painting. That fall, I noticed more than ever how the leaves smelled in the crisp cool air and how the leaves sounded crunching and crackling under Luke's footsteps and my wheelchair. I liked the way the leaves sounded in the wind, scratching lightly against the pavement. Occasionally, a falling leaf landed on me, and I jumped. I loved the sweet smell of the leaves mixed with the hickory smell of the wood smoke from not too distant fireplaces.

Luke suggested that we go out to a restaurant for a meal. He'd been bringing me back to-go boxes of pizza and hamburgers from my favorite restaurants in town for dinner, but he thought actually going out to eat would be a nice outing. I was afraid everyone would stare at the girl in the wheelchair being fed. But I also wanted a change of scenery, and I missed eating in restaurants.

In October, I finally pushed my misgivings aside—my need to leave my room greater than my fears of being stared at—and Luke and I went out to eat at a Mexican restaurant down the road from the rehabilitation hospital.

My first meal out.

The weather was cool and crisp outside. Not cold at all, but just right. So, we sat at a table outside. A few of my high school friends from field hockey, Jeanie, Lindsey, and Jaclyn, met up with us. The peppery smell of sizzling fajitas wafted out of the restaurant. I ate the nacho chips with my left hand—now my good hand. I had a very hard time carrying out a pinching motion with the fingers in my right hand. I still do. Luke put a handful of chips from the big basket onto a small plate in front of me. I couldn't see well enough and didn't have the coordination to dip them in the salsa, but who needs salsa when you can eat on your own, right?

I didn't look at the menu because I already knew what I wanted: chimichangas!

And I couldn't read the menu. The words just appeared as an assortment of colors through my eyes. I couldn't make out a single word. I knew in my head that there were probably pictures of little tacos and a decorative cactus or two somewhere in this kaleidoscope of color, but I couldn't make anything out.

Luke cut up my chimichangas and fed them to me. Luke wasn't embarrassed or self-conscious in the least to be feeding his wife in a wheelchair. He laughed and smiled, just happy to finally be enjoying dinner at a restaurant with his wife.

We talked about everything, except anything having to do with me being in the hospital. For the first time in a long time, I felt normal. We were the only ones eating outside on the patio. Of course, even if there had been other people around, I wouldn't actually have been able to see them. I wouldn't actually know if they were gawking at the girl in the wheelchair being fed by her husband.

My second outing was to the hair salon. As skilled as Luke became at taming my long curly hair, I decided at the end of October to cut it short. As I re-learned to use my hands more and more, slowly re-mastering fine motor skills, I knew it would be much easier for me to take care of my hair if it was short. If I kept my long hair, I would still need some help if I wanted to take care of it and not constantly look like I'd just rolled out of bed.

Erica, my occupational therapist, took me to a hair salon in Charlottesville. We made an afternoon of it, stopping at Starbucks for lattes afterward. One of my best friends, Jackie, tagged along and snapped a few pictures. The floor to ceiling windows, scent of hair products, and track lighting in the salon provided a welcome change of scenery. I brought a photo my friend Emily found for me in a celebrity magazine to show the stylist what I had in mind.

While she was visiting with me, Emily flipped through a stack of celebrity magazines, trying to find a photograph of someone with a cute haircut. When she told me she found one of Natalie Portman sporting a pixie cut, I said, "Yes! Cut that one out."

I couldn't see the photo, but I could remember

what Natalie Portman's haircut looked like, and that's exactly what I wanted. Some friends asked if I was nervous or if I was sad to cut off all of my beautiful, curly locks. I had never had short hair before, so I was pretty excited.

Someone commented on a photo of my new haircut that Jackie posted shortly afterward on Facebook, saying "I wish I was that brave!" To me it wasn't about being brave. I didn't feel at all nervous or sad. I just felt excited to get a new haircut. I can see how some people might see cutting my hair short as symbolic of the end of a chapter of my life. Honestly, I just saw it as a change I wanted to make. It just made sense. To me it was just a new haircut. Change is not something I've ever been scared of. It also helped that the hairstylist did an excellent job. I didn't quite look like Natalie Portman, but I certainly had a cute haircut. (Luke says I pull it off better than she does.)

For the most part, I felt optimistic about my recovery progress. After I had emerged from my medicated haze and my short-term memory was functioning a little better, I understood what I had to do to get back to being a mommy.

That was my mantra: "I need to get back to being a mommy."

I needed to get stronger and get walking. I needed to first re-learn how to take care of myself (including taking care of my hair), and then I could start re-learning how to take care of my boys.

Being in the rehab hospital gave me a chance to concentrate on getting myself better. I've mentioned that I knew that I had to relearn how to do all of these things. I knew I had to be able to feed myself. I knew I would not be stuck in a wheelchair forever. And I knew I wanted to be able to snuggle with Landon and Parker someday. In light of what I had just been through and all of my doctors' uncertainty about my recovery, how could I have felt so confident I would recover enough to take care of myself and my boys? I don't know how I knew, but I knew.

I never once considered the alternative. I knew that someday, all of these things would happen. Accepting that my brain needed time to heal and not knowing when "someday" would happen was not easy for me. The hardest part was that "someday" wasn't today.

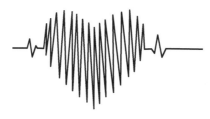

8

One morning, during my first week at the rehab hospital, I awoke to find myself sleeping under a mannequin wearing a wedding dress. When I opened my eyes, I could clearly see layers of white lace and crinoline all around me. Well, I thought that's what I saw, anyway.

The thing was, I wasn't actually seeing anything. It was all a hallucination.

It's not uncommon for people who suddenly lose part of their sight to experience hallucinations. I'm sure all of the strong drugs I took also didn't help: pain medications, heart medications, antibiotics, muscle relaxants, to name a few of the types.

These scenes I thought I saw looked so real; they were crystal clear—much clearer than what I actually saw with my eyes. In those first three weeks at the rehab hospital in August, I didn't really realize the extent of my visual impairment. The hallucinations appeared to be so clear and so frequent that I thought my vision was just fine. That, and being on so much medication, I wasn't entirely clear-headed. Sometimes I just saw an object that wasn't there.

One afternoon, a nurse came into my room, and I asked her "Is that a saddle over there, underneath the TV?"

She said something like "No, no saddles here!"

I knew that I wasn't in a horse stable, and I knew that it didn't make sense for a saddle to be in a hospital room—but I saw it! It looked so real!

Some of the hallucinations I experienced were detailed scenes—incredibly vivid, complete with scents and sounds. In one, Luke and I were nestled in sleeping bags on the floor inside a roadside cafe. Freshly brewed coffee filled my nostrils. The upright metal coffee dispenser gleamed under harsh fluorescent lighting. Everything looked so real!

It seemed odd that we were sleeping in a cafe. I asked Luke, "What are we doing here?"

I thought he must know what was going on. He had no idea either, but he didn't seem to think there was anything strange about the situation. He just shrugged and smiled.

In yet another, Luke and I were dining in a

magical tree house. While we were eating our dinner in this beautiful, enchanted restaurant, Luke let out a loud, rip-roaring belch.

"Luke!" I gasped. "How could you be so rude? There are other people here trying to enjoy their dinner!" Luke didn't seem to understand. He didn't even put down his fork; he just kept on eating.

Most of my hallucinations were strange but not at all frightening. The last one that I remember, however, was pretty morbid. In it, my mother was pushing my wheelchair down the hall back to my room after a physical therapy session. Ahead of me, I saw dismembered body parts hanging all along the left wall of the hallway. Plastic lined the walls, and the plastic was smeared with what looked like fresh blood. It reminded me of cuts of meat hanging in the window of a butcher's shop, except these were clearly human body parts. I casually mentioned it to my mother, as if I was commenting on the hospital's choice of wallpaper.

"Mom, I know it's not real, but it looks like there's body parts on the walls. There are legs, arms, a neck and shoulders, and they're all bloody." I wasn't really freaked out at the time. I knew the strange images I thought I saw weren't real. If my mother was freaked out, she didn't show it.

I think she said something like, "Mmm, that's interesting. But there are definitely no body parts on the walls."

After the hallucinations stopped happening, I started working on vision exercises with my occupational therapist, Erica. During the first sessions of therapy, I sat at a table, and Erica said to me "Tell me what numbers are on these playing cards."

It wasn't that I had trouble reading the numbers on the cards; I didn't even *see* any playing cards fanned out on the table at all. I was dumbfounded. *Wow*, I thought to myself, *there is something very wrong with my vision.*

Up until this point, I hadn't been asked to focus on anything. My surroundings were blurry, but that didn't bother me too much. When I was in the coma, the doctors told my family blindness was a certainty. Compared to being blind, blurry vision really didn't seem so bad. Of course, I hoped that my vision would get better on its own with time or that maybe some kind of eye surgery or glasses would help, but I could deal with blurry vision. However, when I realized that I simply couldn't see the playing cards—objects that were right in front of me—I knew something was really wrong.

Confused, I told her "I can't see any cards."

Erica knew just what to do. "Let's forget about the numbers right now, and let's work on seeing the cards."

That was all well and good, but I still couldn't see the cards.

Erica didn't give up. Firm and patient, Erica told me, "Just keeping looking."

"I really can't see them at all."

"Keep looking Carolyn."

I took a deep breath and tried to keep focussing on the table in front of me. Suddenly, I caught a glimpse of something that looked like a card, but just as suddenly as the card had appeared, it disappeared. "Wait, wait, I saw something, but now it's gone."

"Good, just keep looking and it will come back. I'm going to hold up a single card, and you need to tell me what color it is. Is it red or black?"

After a few minutes, the card came into focus again. Before I had finished saying "It's red," the card had disappeared.

To make it easier, Erica swapped the playing cards for sheets of brightly colored construction paper. The sheets of paper were bigger and easier to focus on, for starters. She held a sheet of paper directly in front of my face, about two feet away.

"Pink," I said.

But when Erica moved the piece of pink construction paper even slightly to my left or right, I couldn't see it. This was the first hint that my peripheral vision might be compromised. I'd have to see a specialist, a neuro-ophthalmologist, to determine what exactly was going on with my vision.

Erica and I worked on reading the numbers on the cards the following session. Again, Erica held up a playing card and asked me to tell her what number I saw on it. And again, I couldn't see the card.

"When you can see the card, look in the upper left corner. You know that's where the number is," Erica instructed.

It took a while for me to be able to read the number. At first, the card would come into view. Then, it disappeared too quickly for me to be able to make out the number. Eventually, I trained my eyes to move in order see the number.

"Five! It's a five!" I said, surprised I was able to see it, even if it was just for a second.

These exercises slowly became less difficult for me as my vision improved. After several weeks of working on this exercise, I could identify the suit of the card— whether it was a ten of spades or a ten of hearts.

Erica stripped down the exercise to its most basic parts: the color of the card, the number of the card, and the suit of the card. By working with me on each of these parts individually, one at a time, Erica was able to shift my focus from what I couldn't see in order to help me find what I could see. She pushed me, but Erica also broke things down into manageable pieces. Instead of working on numbers when I couldn't even see the cards, Erica and I worked on identifying colors. Colors I could do. Erica helped me find the cards in the scrambled picture that I saw as the world.

To me, the world looked like an old television stuck on a channel that wasn't working, what some people call snow. Everything looked grainy. But besides things just being blurry, I had trouble focusing on things. That was always the trouble: finding things in my field of vision. Focusing on one thing was difficult. Focussing on more than one thing at the same time seemed almost impossible. When I concentrated on looking at one spot, eventually an object would materialize. But once something appeared in my field of vision, it only remained there momentarily. Just as suddenly as it had appeared, the object suddenly dissolved into the static. All that was left was a fuzzy TV screen.

Relearning how to focus on objects in front of me was like looking at pictures in a Magic Eye book. The instructions in the front of the book tell you to hold the page with the picture to your nose and then slowly move it away. The instructions say not to look *at* the image, but *through* the image, and wait for it to appear. In a similar way, the actual act of seeing for me was like looking at a Magic Eye picture—there were steps that I had to learn and follow in order to see the image. And Erica helped me figure out and learn to follow those steps.

As I mentioned earlier, Erica was my occupational therapist. Strictly speaking, working on my vision was outside of her role as an occupational therapist. Erica's primary role was to help me relearn how to do daily tasks. She taught me how to fold clothes, dress myself, set the table, and shower all by myself. Erica dedicated our therapy time to helping me become independent so that I could get back to raising my family. Erica really understood how important it was to me to get back to being a mommy as soon as possible.

But working on improving my vision also fell outside the roles of my physical therapist and my speech therapist—meaning that working on my vision wasn't on the agenda at all. But Erica went above and beyond. Not only did Erica take me out to get my haircut in Charlottesville, but she also even came out to visit with me after I left the rehab hospital. Erica helped me out with a few things I struggled with, namely getting some of my clothes on.

Erica's mother had experienced similar vision problems. So, my vision problem was an issue close to her heart. I think the general consensus by most of the health professionals at the rehab hospital in regards to my sight was to wait and see. My records said that I was blind; end of story. My vision would either get better on its own, or it wouldn't. Erica felt a more proactive approach was best. This was why she developed a number of eye exercises for me.

Our personalities really clicked, and Erica and I became close. Erica was motivated, enthusiastic, and direct. When I had trouble seeing something during the vision exercises, she said "Just look at it." She helped me refocus my mind, which was essential for relearning how to focus my eyes.

The vision exercises I worked on with Erica revealed definite problems with my peripheral vision, but the extent of the problems weren't clear. At the time, articulating the nature of my visual impairments was difficult. To figure out what exactly was going on with my vision, I needed to see a specialist for testing. Erica worked on getting me an appointment with a world-renowned, neuro-ophthalmologist, Dr. Robinson. She phoned his office every day for weeks, asking if there had been any cancellations.

In the meantime, my psychologist started doing some simple testing at the rehab hospital. He drew some pictures on a white board—four easily recognizable objects: A house, a tree, a cloud, and a sun.

"What do you see Carolyn?" he asked.

"A house," I said, feeling reasonably confident and pleased that I was able to correctly identify an object. This was good! Things were starting to look up. I could just make out the shapes, a triangle on top of a square. A house.

"Good, what else do you see?"

What? There were more pictures? Where?

"Um, nothing...I just see a house," I said

The house had been drawn in the middle of the board; the tree on the left side; the cloud in the upper left corner; and the sun in the upper right corner. The evidence of my responses suggested that my peripheral vision was significantly compromised. I could see the house because it was in the very center of the white board, directly in front of me.

My psychologist instructed me to shift my gaze to the left.

"Now what do you see?" he asked.

I didn't see anything at first. A few moments later, a drawing of a tree materialized out of the static. But the moment I shifted my gaze just ever so slightly to the left, the house vanished.

The white board wasn't exactly massive, so each of these drawings couldn't have been more than a few inches apart. I had extreme tunnel vision.

Not being able to see well made everything in physical and occupational therapy more difficult, but it also tried my emotions. I hated that I couldn't *see* Landon and Parker when they came to visit.

Landon's second birthday was especially difficult. At the end of August, we threw a small birthday party in the hospital cafeteria with family and close friends. It was in the evening, so we had the place to ourselves. My mother sat next to me and narrated, describing each present as Landon unwrapped it. I didn't need to see Landon to know he was excited and happy. I heard the enthusiasm in Landon's voice. I heard Landon laughing. I heard the bell on Landon's new tricycle as he zoomed around the cafeteria. But I hated that I couldn't *see* the look on Landon's face as he unwrapped each of his presents. I couldn't *see* Landon's smile or the way Landon's eyes must have lit up with the discovery of each new delight.

This was not how I envisioned Landon's second birthday party. I was at my son's birthday party, but I wasn't part of it. Not in the way that I thought I should be. I sat on the side-lines. I felt like I was only an observer, a spectator. I wasn't *being* his mother. I wasn't handing him birthday presents or slicing the cake or running around checking if everyone had everything they needed.

I'm a planner. I love planning things like birthday parties. I love picking out matching invitations, party favors, and decorations. For Landon's first birthday a year ago, everything was Curious George. We bought a Curious George birthday cake for him and sent out Curious George themed invitations. I wasn't happy. I was missing an opportunity to plan my sons' second birthday. (This one would have been Diego themed. That was his new favorite show.)

But I was happy to *be* there, despite my vision impairment.

Reading and writing were two other things that I needed to completely relearn. Aside from not being able to *see* the letters, I couldn't *remember* how to use a pencil to form any letters. It was as if I'd never been able to write. I could still recognize letters and numbers. If I saw a letter M, I knew it was a letter M, and I knew what sound it made. I could recognize letters when I could make them out, but seeing the letters was difficult.

My speech therapist, Mallory, helped me relearn to read and write. I started off learning to write before I learned to read again. Learning to read again came later, and it came much slower than learning to write—mostly because of the extent of my visual impairments.

Mallory and I both knew that holding a pencil was going to be a challenge in and of itself, but the first step would be to teach me the letters. I'm glad Mallory knew where to start, because I certainly didn't. The simple part of forming the letters was difficult for me. Children gradually work up to writing. They watch adults and older children do it. They watch their mothers hold a pen and make a list, their kindergarten teacher hold chalk to draw letters on the chalkboard. While it's difficult for children in the beginning, they catch on fast, because they see it constantly going on around them. But I had to relearn the whole writing process all over again, as if for the first time.

Mallory thought the best way to teach me letters was to break everything down, so that I only had to deal with one challenge at a time. First, I started tracing letters with my finger. Mallory guided my hand, as I traced letters on the table with my pointer finger.

We decided to focus first on only uppercase letters. That meant learning 26 characters, as opposed to 52, if I would've tried to learn both lower and uppercase. I could get by knowing how to write just uppercase letters.

Lots of people write in all capital letters. Writing in all lowercase letters, however, just isn't done. And there's a reason kids learn to write uppercase letters before they learn their lowercase letters. Uppercase letters are easier to tell apart from each other. (Remember how confusing those lowercase letters b and d in elementary school were?) And uppercase letters are simply easier to write.

If I could write uppercase letters, I could write words, and then, sentences. I could be able to effectively communicate on paper. I could learn the lowercase letters another day, sometime down the road. (To this day, though, I still cannot write lowercase letters. I guess that speaks to how well knowing only capital letters has served me.)

After a little practice writing letters, Mallory and I started practicing on numbers. I did the same thing that I did to learn letters. I started out tracing numbers on the table with my pointer finger. Then, I drew the letter or number in the air. Finally, I started writing letters and numbers out with a pencil. Every night in bed before I went to sleep, I'd trace letters and numbers with my finger in the air. I wanted to make sure I remembered them all.

Once I knew my uppercase letters and my numbers again and could trace each one with my finger in the air, Mallory and I moved on to learning to hold a pencil. I was excited to actually start writing again. Of course, like relearning everything else, holding a pencil felt incredibly unnatural, just as it probably does to children when they are switching from big crayons to pencils.

At first I held the pencil with my fist, the same way that I held my fork. Just like a toddler. I'm right-handed, so it didn't help that the right side of my body was most affected by the brain damage. The pencils I used were all outfitted with rubber grips, to make holding them a little bit easier. Every time I picked up the pencil, Mallory had to help me correctly position my fingers and explain what she was doing each time.

"Grip the pencil with your thumb and forefinger and let it rest on your middle finger," she'd tell me.

Very deliberately, I moved each individual finger into place. I drew shaky lines across the paper with the pencil, but I did not draw letters. I wasn't able to write letters for several months after I came home from the rehab hospital. This was something I finished learning while going to outpatient therapy.

Around the same time that I learned to recognize the suits of the playing cards during occupational therapy sessions, Mallory and I started working on teaching me to learn to read again. She spent several weeks working with me to help me learn to identify letters on a page. Mallory would draw three large letters on the board in uppercase, since I hadn't relearned lowercase letters.

Mallory always made sure to leave enough space between the letters. If they were too close together, they blurred together. My brain needed as much simplicity as possible. Reading just a single letter proved extremely difficult in the beginning. Just like seeing any other object, I waited until the letter emerged from the static in my vision. Usually, the letter remained in my field of sight long enough for me to recognize the letter, but the letter soon disappeared back into the static. Since my brain could only process one letter at a time, reading entire words— let alone sentences—was impossible for the time being. I needed to give my brain more time to heal.

Besides the occasional celebrity magazine, I was never much of a reader, but I needed to be able to help teach Landon and Parker how to read and write. I needed to be able to read to send emails, to help the boys with their homework, and to make grocery lists. I needed to be able to read bills that came in the mail and newsletters and hand-outs that the kids brought home from school. The list just goes on and on.

These were the things I always thought about that motivated me to keep going with therapy and rehabilitation. I had to take things one step at a time. I'd be overwhelmed if I tried to relearn everything all at once. I kept reminding myself that it would still be a few years until either Landon or Parker would need to learn how to read. Landon was the oldest, and he was only two. So, I had at least a couple years until Landon would start learning to read.

My vision improvement was slow. I was eager for my appointment with Dr. Robinson, the brain-eye specialist. I hoped there might be some kind of procedure or even corrective glasses that could help my vision improve. Erica managed to book an appointment for me in September. She warned me that Dr. Robinson had a reputation. He didn't have the best bedside manner, she cautioned. But he was one of the very best in the neuro-ophthalmology field.

Sure enough, Dr. Robinson reminded me of a mad scientist right from the start of the appointment. His speech was pressured and quick. I heard him pacing around the room as he spoke. Dr. Robinson performed several tests. In between each test, he muttered something while furiously scribbling away on a pad of paper, and then he abruptly left the room.

First, he asked me to read an eye chart. I couldn't read a single letter, not even the big E at the top. *This is bad*, I thought.

Next, he shined a bright light in my eyes, asking me to move my eyes left and right.

After that, he had me sit in a little dark room and hold a trigger of some sort in my hand. Dr. Robinson told me to squeeze the trigger whenever I saw a bright light out of the right or left side of my peripheral vision.

Nothing.

I didn't see a single flash of light cross in my line of vision. My peripheral vision was bad, but I didn't realize how bad.

In that dark room with my face pressed up against the screen, I started to feel hopeless. How was I going to take care of Landon and Parker if I could hardly see? How was I going to know if they were playing too close to the road? How was I going to keep them out of danger?

The results of the tests were not good, just as I suspected.

"There is nothing that can be done as far as surgery or any other procedure that would help get back your eyesight. It's possible some of the sight may return, but only time will tell," Dr. Robinson said.

Time did tell. As my vision slowly improved, I could focus better on objects. Gradually, the quick glimpses I caught of objects in front of me lasted longer and longer before they disappeared. Eventually, they quit disappearing, and I no longer had to concentrate to see things in front of me.

By the beginning of October, I could almost see well enough to identify objects that were up to five feet away from me. I could see someone's face if he or she was positioned close enough to my line of vision, blurry but recognizable.

Recognizing who a face actually belonged to, however, was an issue. It wasn't a problem for people I saw often, like Luke and frequent visitors, like Slade and Luke's uncle. But it was an issue for people that I didn't see quite so often. I was still good at recognizing voices, so I usually got by.

When friends from my old field hockey team organized a benefit for me, I really worried about not being able to recognize people. We expected a lot of people to show up. There's no way I'd recognize everyone. People have trouble putting a name to a face, from time to time. For me, it was like that constantly.

There is actually a specific part of the brain that is devoted to recognizing human faces. And that part of my brain had been damaged. To my relief, people were incredibly understanding. Luke and my friends that organized the event did a great job of letting people know that I had trouble recognizing faces. Almost everyone introduced themselves when they approached me, to my relief.

The benefit was held at the football stadium at James River High School, where we used to play field hockey. It started out as just a field hockey alumni game. As more people became involved, it grew into a huge carnival. Eventually, my field hockey teammates formed a planning committee to delegate tasks. There were bands, t-shirts, auctions, games, food stands, and even two bounce houses—those giant inflatable castles that kids can jump around in.

In the past, we had hosted these kinds of benefits for other people. Never in a million years did I think a benefit would be put on for me! Slade was instrumental in putting the word out there and getting the committee started.

The local news announced the event and explained my story. They interviewed me a couple days before the event, on the back patio of the hospital. I was so nervous! My short-term memory was not great at that point, so I was scared I was going to lose my train of thought mid-sentence during the interview. To my surprise, I didn't make any mistakes.

The turnout at the benefit was incredible. After hearing my story, people that didn't even know me contributed their time and money to the event. All in all, $23,000 was raised.

Everyone gathered together in the way that people usually only do for weddings or funerals. Friends from my high school years, former teachers and coaches, family, friends of friends, nurses from both the ICU in Richmond and the rehab hospital at UVA, and even the paramedics that restarted my heart and brought me to the hospital showed up at the event.

People came from as far away as Texas. They were all completely shocked at how far I'd come. I definitely felt a renewed sense of strength, knowing there were so many people cheering me on.

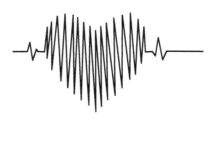

9

Coming to terms with the ways that my brain had been affected by the lack of oxygen happened little by little. I realized how bad my vision was when I couldn't see the playing cards that Erica had asked me to identify on the table. When Mallory asked me to tell her my address and Parker's middle name, I couldn't. I realized, then, that my short term memory was bad. I realized just how much my brain had been changed since I started physical therapy. None of my organs or muscles were damaged. Only my brain was damaged, but it affected my entire body.

The short-circuiting of the neurons in the damaged parts of my brain made movement very difficult for a variety of reasons. The main reasons for these difficulties were that my brain wasn't effectively communicating with my muscles. As a

Carolyn Powell

result, my balance was very poor.

In order to learn to walk, I needed to learn to stand. My physical therapist, Theresa, started with balance assessments. When asked to stand up straight for my first few balance assessments, I thought my posture was standing up stick-straight. I remember feeling wobbly and thinking that my strength wasn't what it should be, but I thought I was standing up straight. Theresa told me that my body actually leaned about 20 degrees to the left.

Watching yourself in a full-length wall mirror can be helpful in correcting posture. Most patients with my issues used that approach, but this wasn't an option for me, because of my blurry vision. At this point, my vision was so scrambled that I still had trouble identifying simple shapes. Making sense of my leaning posture in the mirror was impossible. I had to rely on my therapists' words and hands, shifting me into an upright position, to work on my posture.

I was determined to walk again, but I was up against a lot of obstacles: poor balance, muscle weakness, muscle stiffness, and brain damage. The parts of my brain responsible for movement were very damaged. As a result, I had major problems making my body move the way I wanted it to. That was the biggest obstacle.

This was going to be a challenge—and I was up for it. I had nothing to lose and everything to gain.

By the end of August, I had been at the rehab hospital for a month. Parker was working on getting from his tummy to a crawling position. I never imagined that my infant son and I would learn to walk at the same time. Parker started off raising himself up on his elbows. After he had that down, he raised himself up on his elbows and started squirming around, moving, but not getting very far. A couple months later, he could get up on his hands and knees and gradually started to crawl.

The process I went through to relearn how to walk was very much the same: it was gradual, and it was all about balance. Working on the floor mats, I was supposed to push myself from either a seated or lying position onto all fours, but I couldn't do it at first. It took two weeks for me to build up enough strength to raise myself from my stomach onto all fours. Once I got onto my hands and knees, I felt incredibly unsteady.

Once we've mastered crawling and walking as young children, it's hard to imagine either of these movements being difficult. It seems hard to imagine feeling unstable while balancing on your hands and knees, but my balance was so bad and my muscles were so weak, that—even on all fours—I felt like I was going to topple over at any moment.

Being able to get onto all fours is one of the easiest ways to get from a sitting position on the floor to a standing position. When people fall, this is usually how people get up. For a long time, that wasn't something I was able to do. That was one of the reasons I became so afraid of falling—I couldn't get back up again on my own.

Figuratively, I was great at falling and getting right back up again. I've always had the determination to overcome obstacles in my path, such as being told I'd be confined to a wheelchair the rest of my life. Literally falling and getting back up again was a different story. Despite months of physical therapy, my body still didn't know how to fall.

Falling typically causes reflexes to kick in. Arms immediately extend and certain muscles contract to minimize injury because that is the typical, reflexive response from a body falling. The imperfect way my muscles and brain communicated didn't allow for this reflexive type of response.

I felt like I didn't remember how to fall. When I did fall, I fell over like a tree being cut down in a forest. My body did nothing to minimize injury. So not only did I feel like I was going to topple over anytime I was on my feet because I was so unsteady and weak, I was afraid that if I did fall, I would get hurt.

In some ways, my experience learning how to walk again differed from Parker's experience learning to walk for the first time. Watching a baby learning to walk for the first time is usually an exciting and happy experience for everyone involved. Despite falling every few steps, smiles and giggles celebrate this learning milestone for children.

I remember when Landon first learned to walk, not so long ago. Like most kids, he just took a couple steps, wobbled, and then fell. Sometimes he fell forward and caught himself with his little hands, and sometimes he toppled backward and landed on his bottom. Either way, he almost always caught himself, landing un-phased. Landon got right back up on his feet to try it again.

Babies aren't afraid of falling when they're walking. I don't know for sure why that is, but I think it might have something to do with their distance from the ground. They are close to the ground, so they really don't have far to fall. Chances are good that they won't get hurt. At five-foot–eight-inches tall, I had much farther to fall than

Landon or Parker. More scary, I didn't know how to fall anymore.

Learning how to walk again was a terrifying experience. It's one of the scariest things I've ever done. For me, fear entirely eclipsed the joy of my first steps. Taking my first steps with the walker terrified me. Falling still terrified me much later, when I took my first steps without my walker. As much as I wanted to walk on my own again, I couldn't shake my fear of falling. I've never actually walked across a rickety wooden bridge stretching over a deep rocky canyon, but that's the fear I associated with walking across a room.

With the aid of a walking machine, a treadmill with robot components, I took my first steps on August 7th, two weeks after I arrived at the rehab hospital. The robotic treadmill and three therapists—Mallory, Erica, and Theresa—did most of the work. I just hung from the equipment like a marionette puppet, scared of falling. My therapists wanted to get me upright as soon as possible. Strapping me into the walking machine helped them determine how close, or how far, I was to walking again.

Each session using the walking machine only lasted about ten minutes, but it always felt much longer. Mallory, Erica, and Theresa strapped me into a harness and suspended my body over a treadmill in an upright position. This complicated looking harness worked to reduce the amount of body weight that my legs needed to support during my walk. Both the harness and the robotic component stabilized my body. My ankles and legs were strapped into a robotic component of the machine that actually moved my legs in a walking motion. I was thoroughly strapped in and encased in various safety harnesses, but I held tight to the treadmill bars, feeling unsteady as a rag doll. Even strapped into all of this equipment, I was terrified of falling.

After each ten-minute session, my hands ached for hours from gripping onto the treadmill bars too tightly. My movements were jerky and my steps, heavy. I felt like I had little control over my movements, like a marionette puppet in the hands of an unskilled puppeteer—me. I walked lopsided, throwing my weight to the left, my "good" side. I couldn't believe how unnatural walking felt. I felt as if I'd never done this before, even though I had walked for 27 years before my cardiac arrest. I had hoped that it was being in a robotic walking machine that made walking feel unnatural to me, but when I finally started taking cautious steps with my walker, it still felt unnatural.

As luck would have it, the clinic was producing a commercial to trot out all of their brand new therapeutic equipment. The walking machine was truly the most prized of all the new equipment. Consequently, they wanted substantial footage of this particular machine being put to good use.

I like to think they selected me for the role of "walking machine user" because of my impressive acting resume. In my early twenties, I modeled fur coats in commercials for the local furrier. These were mostly aired during Christmastime and featured me and about three other models sporting the latest in mink coats and ermine stoles, laughing, smiling, and trying our best to look fetching. Personally, I think we looked ridiculous, but if that's what sells fur coats, then so be it. I'm quite certain it's also what got me this gig.

The general idea while making a commercial is to make people think that the product will make users happy. Just as this was the goal of the local furrier in town, this was also the goal of the rehab hospital. The man working the camera asked if maybe Theresa and I could conjure up some laughs and smiles—make it look like loading me into and walking in a harness (like Pinocchio when he had strings) constituted a good time.

Theresa knew that I was *not* having a good time. Not falling required all of my energy and focus. There was none left for fake laughing, so Theresa asked me to tell her a joke or say something funny. Without missing a beat, I told her to imagine how hot we both looked right then—her holding my harness and me leaning slightly to the left. Theresa lost it, and she couldn't stop laughing for a solid ten minutes.

After a few sessions in the walking machine, it was clear that I wasn't quite ready to start walking on my own. I had been lying in a hospital bed for four weeks, so I'd lost a lot of strength. My balance was totally off. I'd have to take a few steps back first, and start with the basics.

Early on, I managed to stand for brief periods of time. First, I stood for ten minutes. A week later, I stood for twenty minutes. Standing in place completely exhausted me.

For most of the month of August and into September, I spent most of my time during physical therapy sessions working at a set of parallel bars on my balance. For these exercises, I held on to the parallel bars while standing on a balance board or a foam ball.

These exercises reminded me of practicing lifts in synchronized swimming. There are three different positions for the swimmers involved in a typical lift. When I practiced synchronized swimming, one girl floated face down in the water while one girl stood on top of her, and five girls positioned underneath the middle girl. The girls at the bottom of the arrangement did eggbeaters to propel themselves upward, simultaneously pushing the middle girl towards the surface of the water. The girl on the top had to crouch down until her head broke the surface, and then this girl had to quickly rise to a standing position. One of her feet balanced on the middle girl's lower back, and the other on the middle girl's upper back. If the top girl's feet were too far apart she'd tip over, and if her feet were too close together, she'd tip over. The girl in this position needed to have a great deal of balance, and that girl had always been me.

Another activity my therapist had me work on in the beginning was pivoting from my wheelchair to a raised mat. I kept swinging my butt in the wrong direction. It was the same story if I tried to get from the raised mat back to the wheelchair. I always moved in the opposite direction that I intended to move. I never quite got the hang of it. I sometimes wonder if I never got it because I knew it wasn't something I needed to know how to do. It was a useful exercise to get from the wheelchair and into bed, but I didn't plan to sit here for long. I had no desire to waste my energy honing my wheelchair skills, because I was not going to be in a wheelchair for much longer. I didn't care how scary walking felt. I was going to do it.

When the day finally arrived for me to start walking with the walker, I was almost more excited than nervous. It was mid-October. Yes, the walking itself terrified me, but making progress made me so happy that my happiness overshadowed my terror. As I took those first cautious little steps with the walker, I felt for the first time that I really was going to be able to live a normal life. My strength and balance had improved, even though I still felt incredibly unsteady. Theresa and another therapist walked right beside me, holding me up with a thick, cloth belt around my waist, to help them catch me if I fell.

After a week of practicing in the therapy room, we took to the halls.

Before I could leave the rehab hospital, I had to be able to walk on my own with a walker down one of the hallways from the therapy room to the nurses' station and back. While it still seemed daunting, I knew I was getting closer to that goal. For a little while, it felt like things moved along at a good pace. Two weeks after I started using the walker, I started having issues with my balance again. I felt so frustrated—I'd been practicing and I'd been making such great progress. Was I not going to get any better than this? Why was this happening? What had changed?

Theresa didn't seem too concerned. She thought that the muscle spasticity combined with my anxiety made my muscles stiff and had helped me to stand up so straight. Now that the muscle spasticity subsided and I felt a little more steady and relaxed, I was off-center again.

Standing, walking, and other simple movements that most people seldom think about actually take a lot of complex brain activity to happen. It's like seeing, something most people take for granted. People who can see don't think about seeing; they just do it. But there are a lot of things that need to happen in the brain for people to be able to see and for the brain to translate the knowledge of what is seen.

All of the brain activity involved in standing and walking movements take place in certain parts of the brain: the premotor cortex, the motor cortex, the cerebellum, and the basal ganglia. Except for my cerebellum, all of these other parts of my brain were damaged. Since all of these parts of the brain work together in order for me to move, it's no wonder I had trouble walking.

The parts of the brain that control movement in a person's body are part of what's called the motor system. It's a collection of interconnected nerve and muscle cells, extending from the brain, down into the spine, and through our muscles. The motor system controls body movement. Each part of the brain involved in the motor system has a different role in the process of making each part of the body move. One part of the brain is responsible for planning and executing movements. Another part of the brain is in charge of storing learned movements—like riding a bike and walking—and another part of the brain is responsible for coordination. All of these parts work together to make the motor system function. My motor system had sustained significant damage.

The human brain is simultaneously incredibly resilient and incredibly fragile. Until recently, scientists thought that only young children's brains were capable of forming new connections between neurons. Consequently, scientists thought that the loss of functions as a result of damage to an adult brain resulted in permanent function loss.

Recent research indicates that this isn't the case. The human brain has the ability to form new connections between neurons in response to injury or damage. This ability is called neuroplasticity. Neuroplasticity can be a difficult concept to fully grasp. It took me awhile to fully understand. Even after I felt like I had a good understanding of the concept, I had a lot of trouble explaining it to other people. In an audiobook I listened to called *My Stroke of Insight*, brain scientist Jill Bolte Taylor gives a great analogy explaining how neuroplasticity works:

> *I think of the brain as a playground filled with lots of little children. All of these children are eager to please you and make you happy...You look at the playground and note a group of kids playing kickball, another acting like monkeys on a jungle gym, and another group hanging out by the sandbox. Each of these groups of children are doing different yet similar things, very much like the different sets of cells in the brain. If you remove the jungle gym, then those kids are not going to just go away, they are going to mingle with other kids and start doing whatever else is available to be done. The same is true for neurons. If you wipe out a neuron's genetically programmed*

function, then those cells will either die from lack of stimulation or they will find something new to do.

Several of my therapists recommended this book. *My Stroke of Insight* is a memoir, chronicling Jill Bolte Taylor's recovery from a stroke she experienced. As a brain scientist, her knowledge of the brain and how it works gave her a unique insight into her own recovery experience.

I didn't have a stroke, but there are definite similarities between recovering from a stroke and recovering from a brain injury like mine. Both involve dealing with the death of brain cells. I could really relate to certain parts of her experience as she describes them in the book. Her explanation of neuroplasticity really resonated with me. It was easy to understand. Her analogy comparing neurons responding to a brain injury and children doing different activities on a playground made it easy for me to visualize the way that neuroplasticity works.

It's really amazing that to this day, the human brain is still such a mystery. When I was admitted to the intensive care unit, the doctors didn't know what was going to happen. Even with the aid of state of the art medical technology, the doctors had no idea what outcomes would result from my recovery (or lack of recovery). And what conclusions they did draw—that I would be completely blind and most likely a vegetable—were completely upended by my recovery.

The possibility that comes with uncertainty both gave me hope and left me frustrated. I hated having no timeline to map out my recovery, but the possibility that I'd make a significant recovery existed – and that made me happy.

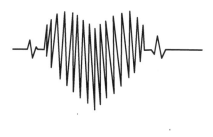

10

Not being able to move like I used to was getting old. Every movement challenged me; everything I did frustrated me. I missed doing things like taking showers, walking, frying eggs, and using a fork to eat—without help. I missed lifting Landon over my head and watching him coo with delight in my own arms. I missed running with Luke. And I missed not having to think about these things.

Therapy exhausted me. I didn't even remember feeling this tired during field hockey, synchronized swimming, or track practice. Sometimes I felt like I just couldn't go on anymore. But I did. I kept going. During practice, my teammates kept me going. They counted on me. That, and I knew the end result was worth it. The same kind of thoughts got me through rough therapy sessions. Parker and Landon kept me going. They were counting on me, and I knew the end result would be worth it.

My progress in physical therapy was slow, but I learned to celebrate the small victories: when I was able to stand up straight for ten minutes without leaning, I celebrated; and when I was able to lift a medicine ball over my head, I savored a little victory.

In mid-August, after about two weeks at the rehab hospital, I was scheduled for aqua therapy. I was so excited! I knew swimming. This was going to be different than walking.

I knew doing laps as I had once done them wouldn't be on the agenda immediately. I had realistic expectations. I'm driven and compet-itive, but I'm realistic. I would swim maybe a few half laps the first few sessions. They wouldn't be pretty—no butterfly stroke or free style right away. I would have to settle for something closer to a dog paddle. I looked forward to just moving through the water on my own. It wouldn't be pretty, but I was going swimming!

When we arrived at the pool, I caught that sweet familiar scent of chlorine, and my heart soared. Momentarily, I lost myself to memories of my days as a synchronized swimmer. For nine years, my sister Susan and I swam on a synchronized swimming team. I started when I was just nine.

When I say I've always been involved in sports, I really do mean always. Before synchronized swimming, I tumbled in gymnastics. Soon after I started synchro, I also added field hockey and track to the mix. The health club I practiced at was located just down the block from where I lived while growing up, almost in my own backyard.

On most school days, I went to field hockey practice right after school, came home and ate dinner, finished my homework, and went to synchronized swimming practice in the evenings. It was a demanding schedule, but I loved it. I love being busy. (Maybe that is why I've enjoyed being a mother so much?)

I loved the challenge of synchronized swimming. It requires both upper and lower body strength and a lot of coordination. It's not a sport one can just dabble in. It's a difficult sport, but I was a conditioned athlete. I had it all: balance, coordination, strength, and determination. Now, I only had one of those qualities, but that quality—determination—was going to help me get my balance and my coordination back.

While I prepared to get into the rehab pool, I thought back to my days in synchro. My friend,

Lindsey, and I did a duet to the Pulp Fiction soundtrack back in my sophomore year of high school. I could hear the music playing in my mind. Lindsey and I were all decked out in matching sparkly silver bathing suits, our hair up in perfect buns held fast with Knox brand gelatin. The music was fast-paced surf-rock, very high energy.

In the rehab pool, instead of a nose plug and goggles, Theresa and Erica outfitted me with a foam noodle and strapped a flotation belt around my waist. The goal now: to work on staying afloat—not fine tuning a swim routine or practicing breath control. Theresa and Erica guided me into the pool lift, a chair that slowly lowers you into the water.

The chair motor sounded loud and grinding, robotic. As the chair slowly lowered me into the pool, I took in my surroundings. The pool was shallow here, where the chair lowered me into the water. But I wasn't just starting out in the shallow end. There was no shallow end; rather, the entire pool was the shallow end.

Alongside the pool, bins of colorful foam noodles and foam weights and objects lined the walls. Metal handrails ran down the middle of the small pool, presumably for providing balance and carrying out different exercises. This was not the kind of pool for doing laps or synchronized swimming routines. Already, this experience was shaping up to be a far cry from swimming as I'd known it not so long ago.

Being in the water didn't feel good or natural. It felt strange. It wasn't supposed to feel strange. It was supposed to feel good. Walking felt strange, and standing felt strange — couldn't I just have this one thing?

I used to feel graceful in the water. Now, I didn't feel graceful, and I certainly didn't look graceful. Even in the water, my limbs felt unsteady and out-of-control. In the water, the disconnect existing between my brain and my body seemed even more vast.

"Carolyn, I want you to hold on to the side of the pool and slowly kick," Theresa instructed.

I set to work kicking. Well, I thought I was kicking. My brain thought "kick, kick, kick, kick, kick!" But my legs didn't get the message. They moved — in a general sense — but they didn't kick.

To break it down, kicking in the water is a matter of alternating simple leg movements. It was precisely this alternating movement that my brain had trouble processing. My legs could only manage uncoordinated movements, like how a turtle's legs move around strangely when it has been suddenly

Carolyn Powell

tipped on its back. These movements would have done nothing to prevent me from sinking to the bottom of even this shallow pool.

Even with the flotation belt secured around my waist, my hips dipped well below the surface of the water. Theresa gently but firmly lifted my hips up so that they were just below the surface of the water. I felt a hot lump in my throat. This was supposed to be easier. Being able to swim was supposed to be the one thing I could still do, and I didn't even have that.

Theresa continued instructing me to kick. If she was disappointed in my progress, her voice didn't betray it. Gradually though, she offered easier exercises. Her voice remained encouraging and never wavered. We tried exercises alternating my arms and moving them above my head, and those were a little easier to do, but it felt like only a small consolation.

The only thing I could do was to have faith in my therapists and in myself and just keep working. I needed to keep attempting to carry out the simple commands until my brain relearned how to properly communicate with my body. For now, swimming was just like the rest of my physical therapy: slow-going, hard work.

In synchronized swimming, field hockey, and track, the harder I practiced, the better I got. I know that doesn't seem terribly remarkable; after all, that is the whole idea of practice, to become better at whatever it is you're practicing doing. The rewards I reaped as an athlete were very immediate. I got a rush from mastering skills in sports through practice, and most things came pretty easily. I don't remember any moves in any of the sports I played that I simply couldn't do.

I remember learning how to do an eggbeater. An eggbeater is a basic kick used in synchronized swimming to tread water. The back is straight and both legs are in a sort of seated position, with both thighs parallel to the surface of the water. Keeping the back straight, move the right leg in clockwise circles, and move the left leg in counter clockwise circles. It takes a lot of coordination. Mr. Day, my coach, only showed me once, and I got it. Just like that. I didn't go home that evening until I felt like I could do it. My eggbeaters weren't perfect the first day I started doing them, but I had the basic movements down. I had the coordination. I had the strength. It was only a matter of refinement.

Practicing in rehab was different because I didn't have the coordination. I didn't have the strength. I started off not being able to do anything at all. It wasn't only a matter of perfecting and becoming more proficient at refining things I knew how to do. It was a matter of learning to perform basic movements again from the beginning. I no longer had the strength or the stamina to practice something repeatedly until I got it right.

Sometimes, I'd come away from my therapy sessions frustrated because I felt like I'd accomplished nothing. It took a while to get past this, but gradually I realized that by just working hard at physical therapy sessions, I helped my brain to re-establish those lost connections.

By late October, towards the end of my stay at the rehab hospital, I realized that walking wasn't going to get any easier anytime soon. I was making great progress—amazing progress, considering my prognosis when I first arrived at the emergency room at the hospital in Richmond. In the three months I spent at the rehab hospital, I had gone from literally not being able to stand on my own two feet to being able to walk with a walker up and down the halls.

Not only could I not stand when I first arrived here, I couldn't sit up, get myself to the toilet, or use my arms to do anything by myself. I had come a long way. Even though I was getting better at walking, walking didn't feel any easier for me. Walking still felt incredibly unnatural. I still felt very unsteady on my legs, and I was still terrified of falling. I still held on to my walker with an iron grip.

My discharge date had been pushed back a few times, but by October, it was decided that November 7th would definitely be the day. That would be the day as long as I was able to complete the circuit down the hall and back with my walker all on my own.

In the last days of October, I achieved that goal. I was so nervous. I wanted this so bad. I needed to go home and get back to being a mommy to my kids again. As I turned the last corner of the circuit, I felt a rush of excitement—I was almost there! My own rush of excitement threw off my balance, and I almost tipped over. I managed to recover, and I made the circuit!

I was actually really proud that I'd recovered so well from getting thrown off balance. I still couldn't physically get up from falling, but I felt like recovering my balance and continuing on was pretty similar. A small victory celebrated. I was going home.

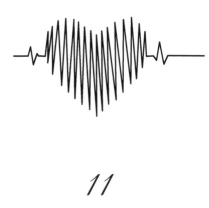

11

Before being discharged from the rehab hospital to go home, Luke and I had to decide where home was going to be. We had absolutely no idea what kind of living situation our family was going to need in the long-term. Was I going to be able to handle stairs eventually? Would we need to find someone to help take care of both me and the boys while Luke was at work?

We didn't know if or when I might get to the point where I could be on my own in the house, let alone take care of Parker and Landon on my own. We didn't know when we were going to know, either. I really thought Luke and I had our lives all figured out until that summer. Up until then, I'd had very few curve balls, good or bad, thrown my way.

I tried to focus on what Luke and I did know. We knew that I was still here, still Carolyn. We knew that Luke, Landon, Parker, and I were all going to live together somewhere as a family. It became clear back in October, after I had been at the rehab hospital for two months, that I wasn't going to need to be in an assisted living care facility for the rest of my life, away from my family. That was such a huge relief for me and for everyone.

During the first few weeks I spent in the ICU, the doctors thought that long-term care would be unavoidable, if I ever even came out of the coma. Me, living out the rest of my days in a long term care facility, blind and unable to communicate in any meaningful way, was the best-case scenario at that point: "She will never be the Carolyn you knew," the doctors told Luke. I wasn't there in the conference room with no windows when the doctors said that, but that statement still echoes in my mind. Not being there to raise Parker and Landon would've broken my heart. I don't think I would've handled being anywhere else very well, without the two most important things in the world to me: my family and my independence. In my mind, that was never an option. I would do whatever it took to get well enough to raise my kids.

My recovery was no doubt miraculous, but it happened at a much slower pace than anyone expected. The rate at which someone recovers from a brain injury is very difficult to predict. It's different for everyone. The three months of intense therapy at rehab had gotten me one my feet. I had made progress for sure. I was hoping to lose the wheelchair for good eventually, but everything was very uncertain. Even with my walker, I still felt very unsteady. I hated being so dependent on it, but at the same time I was still so scared of falling that I couldn't imagine not having it. I worked on regaining the abilities and the strength that I'd lost, but no one really knew what was going to come back and how long it would take. As slow as my recovery seemed, I was still recovering. I was still progressing, and for that, I was thankful.

Because of all the continued uncertainty about how my recovery was going to unfold, we decided to sell the house in Richmond and live at Luke's parents' house, out in Ashland, until the status of my recovery became a little clearer and the boys got a little bit older. Here, Mike and Debbie could help care for both me and the boys.

Living in Ashland at Mike and Debbie's home was exactly what Luke and I needed at the time. Selling our house made sense. I looked forward to a fresh start, but selling our old house was still hard. I was going to miss our old place. It was a three-bedroom Dutch colonial—a smaller version of the house that I grew up in. Luke and I bought the house after a couple years of marriage. I had just finished my dietetic internship, and we were getting ready to start a family. I loved the neighborhood. There were lots of tall pines, and it just felt like home. Luke and I built a brand new deck out in the backyard. The fenced in backyard provided plenty of room for the boys to run but kept them from running too far.

I had spent a lot of time decorating the house, especially the boys' rooms. It seemed like only yesterday that I finished decorating Parker's room. I knew that when we eventually moved out of Mike and Debbie's house, I'd have a whole new house to decorate. I didn't know if my vision would ever be good enough to pick out colors and patterns of curtains, bed spreads, candles, and rugs, but I wanted to think so.

Besides what we brought to Mike and Debbie's— mainly clothes and some of the boys' favorite toys—our things were packed away into boxes in a storage unit. Everything would stay in storage until we were able to embark on the next chapter of our lives, wherever that would be.

When Luke and I moved into his parents' house in November, Landon and Parker were both already settled in. Mike even hung Landon's swing on one of the big oak trees in the Powells' back yard. Landon loved that swing, almost more than his trains. Landon and Parker had been staying with Mike and Debbie since I had been admitted to the hospital, four months prior to Luke and I moving in. Luke had moved Landon's bed and Parker's crib to the house not long after my cardiac arrest, so that Landon and Parker were still able to sleep in their own beds.

Landon's bed—the same bed with the wooden slats on the side where Luke first found me when my heart stopped in July—was in Luke's sister's old room. Parker's crib was at the other end of the hallway, across from Mike and Debbie's bedroom. Luke and I slept in the room next to Landon's.

I missed our house in Richmond, but I was grateful to be welcomed into the Powells' home. Mike and Debbie's help then was absolutely indispensable. They cooked delicious meals for us. They ferried the kids and I around to preschool and therapy and doctor's appointments. I don't know what we would've done without them. I still had some hurdles to overcome.

I struggled getting in and out of Luke's and my

bed. After a few days Luke and I ditched the bed frame and put the mattress on the floor. It was one of the first of many modifications Luke and I made around Mike and Debbie's house to make it easier for me to get around. Sure, Luke was more than happy to help me get in and out of bed, but it was important to me to be able to do it myself.

Next, we put a raised toilet seat with handles over the toilet. A special plastic chair also went into the tiny shower, and we replaced the shower door with a curtain to make it easier for me to get in and out. I wanted to be able to shower in privacy, and I wanted to do it on my own time. I wanted to shower when I wanted to shower. Luke had to help me get in and out, but I could shower on my own by this time. Washing my hair and soaping myself up took much longer than it used to, but I made it work.

Along with all of the medical equipment, Luke and I also bought a big, comfy, reclining armchair for the family room. It was sage green and luxuriously soft, like sitting on a cloud. I wanted to have somewhere that I could nap downstairs so I wouldn't have to go upstairs when Luke was still at work. The chair reclined with a long wooden lever—long enough so I could easily reach it, yet easy for my still weak arms to pull.

Until my brain injury, I had never been one to take naps. Now my body worked overtime, repairing the connections in my brain that had short-circuited and the connections from my brain to my muscles. I grew tired very quickly. As much as I hated sitting still, I knew getting enough rest was essential for recovery. The body repairs itself during sleep, and my body had a lot of repairing to do.

Certain things in the house were easily modified to meet my new needs, like the bed and the bathroom. Others, however, could not be so easily changed. There wasn't anything we could do about the narrow doorways, the hallways, the stairs, and the small size of many of the rooms. It was an old house. A beautiful old house. A Dutch Colonial, like our old house in Richmond. But our old house was only about 30 years old, and the kitchen and bathrooms had all been recently updated. It had an open floor plan that's characteristic of most modern houses. Depending on preference, one might describe old houses like this one as either cramped or cozy. Regardless, we wouldn't live here forever.

One advantage to the narrow hallways and the small rooms were the walls. If I didn't have my walker, there was always a wall within arm's reach on either side of me to steady myself against.

One afternoon, while I made my way back to the living room from the bathroom, my walker tipped over. Normally I would've called out and someone would've given me a hand. That particular afternoon at that particular moment, no one was around. I was very seldom left alone. I felt comfortable being on my own in the house for short periods of time though. I liked it. When my walker went crashing to the ground, I felt a wave of panic, much like whenever I lost my balance momentarily, but worse. I had two options: stand there and be scared and upset and probably fall, or try to make my way back to my chair in the family room. I chose the latter. I balanced myself against the wall and against available edges of sturdy furniture, just like toddlers do when they're cruising during the first stage of learning how to walk. I made it back to my chair without incident that time.

Going through doorways made me anxious. I especially didn't like crossing uneven thresholds. Dividers meant I had to step over something. When there was either a divider along the floor or the floor in one room wasn't quite level with the floor in the adjacent room, I ran into trouble.

When I walked through doorways, I looked down at my feet to make sure my step cleared the threshold. I always stepped right on the threshold because my impaired vision and the disconnected communication between my muscles and my brain caused my depth perception to be slightly off. I always felt like I was going to fall when I stepped onto the uneven flooring in the doorway, but I almost never did.

Luke grew up in this house with his three siblings—two brothers and one sister. Now, the house once again bustled with six people, much as it had when Luke lived here before. Instead of four kids, there were two, but I needed just as much care as a child. So it was like having three. I felt like a child myself. In the beginning, I needed help doing everything.

Being dependent on others was frustrating for me at times, but I knew things would get better. Before I came home to the Powells', the staff at UVA made arrangements for me to continue therapy at an out-patient rehab center with an all-day, month-long program near our old house in Richmond. I started there right away, just two weeks after I left the hospital. The program was all day, from 8:00 a.m. to 5:00 p.m., five days a week. As much as I wanted to spend time at home, I knew how critical time was in my recovery. The more therapy I did early on, the better my chance of recovering as much as possible. And with the Powells' to take care of the boys, this really was the best time to do the program.

Therapy was long, but I ate breakfast and dinner with Landon and Parker and spent time with them in the evenings. That made me happy. Luke was also happy to be home and spending time with his sons. He took over bath time and bedtime stories for the time being.

In the mornings, Debbie made breakfast for Parker, Landon, and I. Luke usually dropped me off at therapy on his way to work. Either Luke's dad, Mike, or one of my friends picked me up from therapy in the afternoon. At all-day therapy, I practiced physical therapy, speech therapy, and occupational therapy, just like I had at the rehab hospital. For the most part I picked up right where I left off.

I always felt like I didn't quite fit in at the out-patient rehab center, though. I was one of the youngest patients by a good thirty years. It felt a little like I was in a retirement center. Most of the therapists themselves were my age, though. A lot of them had children of their own, so they could easily relate to my situation. They knew how important it was for me to become physically independent so that I could get back to taking care of my kids.

There was one other patient my age, relatively speaking. I'll call him Scott. He was in his mid-twenties, about five years younger than me, and in a wheelchair. One night he dove head first into the shallow end of a pool while he was drunk at a party. He hit his head on the concrete bottom of the pool, which left him paralyzed from the neck down.

We talked a lot. We had quite a lot in common: both of us had received a grim prognosis. The doctors had said that if he did wake up from the coma, the best-case scenario for him would be that he'd be in a vegetative state. Both of us had beaten the odds and were doing better than anyone could have dreamed, and we were both motivated to become as independent as possible.

I was touched by Scott's spirit. He had such undying positivity, and he had so much fight in him. Scott was paralyzed, and he hadn't given up, even though he knew his chances of walking ever again were almost non-existent. I had a lot of obstacles before me, but walking was still possible for me. Seeing Scott's motivation first hand put things into perspective for me and fortified my own determination.

My physical therapy routine was much the same as it had been: parallel bars and balance boards. I had progressed, however, to walking without a harness on the treadmill—a normal treadmill, not a puppet-walking machine. I still held onto the side bars with an iron grip, but this time, I did all of the work. I stood up on the belt on my own two feet. I started out walking slowly.

Eventually, my new physical therapist, Jessica, upped the speed by gradual degrees over the course of the session, forcing my brain to keep up with the speed of my legs. A couple weeks into the program, I was able to run on the treadmill for a full six minutes. After that first time running, tired and trying to catch my breath, my hands aching from holding on so tight to the side bars, I felt so good and so proud to achieve another goal. I wasn't sure I still had it in me to run, but I did. I'd come a long way, even though I still had a long way to go to get back to taking care of my boys, but I was getting there.

Just like in speech therapy at UVA, I worked on writing and reading instead of speech at the out-patient rehab center in Richmond. My new speech therapist, Heather, drew three large letters on a white board, but this time the letters formed short words. I moved on from identifying letters to identifying how letters formed words. I read three letter words, at first: cat, sit, bat, and hen.

My brain had healed enough to form new connections that allowed my brain to focus more quickly on each letter. Focusing on individual letters no longer took as much effort as it had before.

Heather taught me how to slowly scan letters from left to right. My gaze was jerky when I scanned. Sometimes my brain skipped over the middle letter, but I could usually figure out the word if I caught the other two letters. I got better and better as the weeks passed. Before the speech therapy program ended, I could even read short sentences: The cat sits on a mat.

I continued to work on relearning to write. I used a marker to write letters on a whiteboard.

In occupational therapy, I worked with my new occupational therapist, Sandra, on strengthening my right hand and working on daily tasks and self-care. My right hand was especially weak and out-of-sync with my brain. I spent a lot of time flipping over coins or bigger round disks.

Erica had worked with me on folding clothes and dressing myself while I was at the rehab hospital, but I still had a long way to go. I continued to work on all of these things at the out-patient rehab center with Sandra.

Folding clothes was still like attempting complicated origami. I didn't know up from down and front from back. Dressing myself was even worse. Each article of clothing required a different strategy. I didn't just need to relearn how to dress myself, I needed to learn how to put on a shirt, how to put on pants, how to put on underwear, how to put on a bra, how to put on socks, and how to put on shoes.

When I first started working on dressing and folding clothes with Erica at the rehab hospital, my vision was terrible. On top of not being able to focus my vision very well, I had little control over the movement of my arms, hands, and legs. This made it difficult to even grasp the technique that involved folding a cloth, much less try to navigate folding a shirt.

I couldn't see well enough to be able to tell which side of a shirt was the front or the back. I couldn't see which end of the shirt was the top or bottom either. I had to use my fingers to feel for the neck opening and the bottom opening. Erica taught me to lay the shirt on my lap so that the neck opening was on my knees. That helped me stay oriented. I still put my shirt on this way now.

"Neck on the knees," Erica would say.

To figure out which side was the front and which side was the back, Erica suggested feeling for clues, like a tag, a tie, or buttons.

"Tie in the front, tag in the back," Erica instructed.

Pants had buttons in the front. When I eventually taught Landon and Parker how to get dressed, I used these same tips.

Erica had plenty of tips and tricks to offer, but a lot of occupational therapy is trial and error. What once worked for me might not work any longer. Even what worked for other people recovering from a similar brain injury wouldn't necessarily work for me.

Before my cardiac arrest, I used to put my shirt on by first putting my head through the neck and then put my arms through the sleeves, but that didn't work for me anymore. After wrestling with my shirt for several sessions with Erica, I finally found a way to make it work. Arms first, one at a time. Then, pull it over my head. It was another six months until I actually mastered my new technique.

Pants were probably the easiest to put on, because it was easy to tell the top from the bottom. The waist was at the top; the legs were at the bottom. All I had to do was feel for the button and the zipper or the tag to know which side was the front and which side was the back.

Putting on underwear was similar to putting on pants but harder. It was difficult for me to feel the difference between the front and the back, and the difference between the leg holes and the waist. Underwear and bras were the most difficult things to get on.

Shoes posed an especially daunting challenge. Which shoe went on the right foot? Which shoe went on the left? I made great strides with getting my shoes on at the out-patient rehab center. Sandra used a black permanent marker to put a mark inside the right shoe where I could see the mark. Once I identified which shoe went on which foot, I had to get them on. Putting on shoes really is a multi-step process. Somehow, I had to negotiate the tongue placement, push my foot all the way into the shoe, and then tie the laces. After a few failed attempts at tying, Sandra and I decided elastic shoelaces were the way to go. Then, I could just pull the elastic tight instead of actually tying the laces.

I practiced setting the table with plastic plates and cups, but I struggled to lay the forks, spoons, and knives down in the correct arrangement. It reminded me of setting my grandmother's table with her good china and good silverware for Christmas dinner. She taught all of her grandchildren (and no doubt her own children) the proper way to set a table. Although I didn't set the table for Christmas dinner myself that year, I was able to hold my fork almost normally at Christmas dinner.

I finished the out-patient therapy program just in time for the holidays—even with staying in the program for an additional two weeks. Both my insurance and the rehab center agreed to let me stay the additional two weeks, since I had made such great progress. I accomplished a lot in out-patient therapy, but I felt like I needed a little more help with some things.

After the holidays were over, I started going to another therapy program at a rehab center closer to the Powells', Hanover Rehabilitation Center. The program was only one hour long, twice a week.

It was nice to spend more time with the boys once I completed all day therapy, but the days were long. My life had taken on a different pace, a much slower pace, and it took a while to get used to. I was used to working and taking care of my kids, always being on the go.

My life has always been fast-paced. Growing

up, I ran from one practice to another, did school work, waited tables at a barbeque restaurant in town, or hung out with friends. College was even more hectic. After college and my internship, my job and my kids kept me very busy. There was never a dull moment, and I loved it.

On the days that Landon attended preschool, getting everyone in the car to take him was a big production. Debbie helped me into the car. She fastened my seatbelt and secured both Landon and Parker in their car seats.

During moments like that, I felt especially like a child. Getting an adult with very limited mobility and a baby in a car is difficult, but it was important to me to be able to take Landon to preschool. Dee-Dee walked Landon into preschool, and I stayed in the car with Parker. It broke my heart to watch them walk in together. I wanted to be the one walking my son into school, but I couldn't. Each day we took Landon to preschool, I'd watch him and his grandmother go through the doors and think will I ever be able to do that?

After we got home from dropping Landon off at preschool, Parker went down for his morning nap. While he slept, I watched TV. It would probably be more accurate to say I listened to the TV. My chair was positioned close to the TV, but my vision could not focus on the picture moving across the screen. In those quiet moments, I practiced walking, folding clothes, and other tasks I worked on in occupational therapy. I practiced some of the exercises that I worked on in physical therapy as well.

I was practicing standing up without using my walker when it happened. As I stood up from my chair, I thought I heard a car pull in the driveway, so I turned my head left. I didn't turn my head especially fast. It was just a glance. I only moved my head slightly, but it was enough to cause me to lose my balance.

My muscles tightened, and my entire body went rigid, stiff as a falling tree. I fell flat on my back, missing the wooden coffee table and the couch by mere inches. Luke heard the crash and appeared there immediately. I only scraped my back a little on the wooden coffee table, but I was rattled. It was the first time I'd fallen since I got back home. After that, I held on even tighter to my walker, and I walked even slower. I stopped practicing standing up unless Luke was nearby to catch me. Sometimes it's one step forward, two steps back.

One thing I started enjoying right away about this slower pace that my life took on was that I now had a lot of time to spend playing with the boys. Spending time with Landon and Parker has always been a priority for me, but I simply didn't have much time before.

When I wasn't at rehab, I got down on the ground with them, amidst a colorful jumble of puzzles, books, blocks, and toy trains, and we played for hours. The toys were very engaging for me. Stacking blocks and trying to put simple puzzles together was incredibly therapeutic for me. Landon was able to put an entire puzzle together by the time I had about three pieces assembled in the right spot on the puzzle I was working on.

Landon loved his trains. They were Thomas the Tank Engine trains, with smiling faces. Each train car had its own name. The name of each train was printed in very small letters on the bottom. Landon liked quizzing me, holding up a train and asking, "Mommy, who is this?"

Percy, Thomas, Edward, Toby, James—I knew the names, but I couldn't see well enough to tell which was which. Even back when I was able to see, I could hardly tell them apart. It seems like all of them are either blue or green.

My experience relearning how to do everything helped me to truly understand the struggles of young children learning to do things for the first time. I could understand where they were coming from.

Learning to dress themselves, feed themselves, catch a ball, and put away their toys is a real challenge. Children have never done any of these things before they do them for the first time. They don't have the muscle memory I had. Developing these skills can be frustrating, especially when other people—the adults in their lives—take these things for granted.

Now that I stayed home with the boys, I was very eager to start trying to do things to help take care of them. I decided to try my hand at bottle-feeding Parker. I missed feeding him. Sitting in my chair, I could hold him in my arms, and I could hold the bottle. I felt like that was a good start.

Actually getting the bottle to Parker's mouth proved to be more difficult than I thought. Parker was close enough to me that I could see his face. It was still blurry, but I could make out his little nose, mouth, and eyes. The problem was my depth perception. That and my muscles still were not in sync with my brain. I kept poking Parker's eye with the bottle.

After about a week, I decided that maybe I

wasn't quite ready to accomplish a bottle feeding with Parker. If I never got the hang of it, that was okay too. Parker wasn't going to be drinking out of a bottle forever. I knew that as Landon and Parker grew, they would need less help with some of the things that were so hard for me now.

Working on the things I needed to learn how to do again to take care of the boys, like feeding them and changing their diapers, was important to me. I didn't know if I was going to be able to do either of those things this early in the game, but I at least wanted to try. I hoped to work on some of these things during therapy.

One day, I packed a diaper and one of Landon's stuffed animals, a duck, in my walker bag—a red tote bag I hung from my walker that served as my purse for the time being. I was excited to try to start working on something that was going to actually help me take care of my boys. I had worked on practicing putting diapers on Landon's stuffed duck with Sandra, but I wasn't very successful. Now, my brain had had more time to heal, so I wanted to give it another try.

When my phase two therapist, Beth, greeted me, I pulled out the diaper and the stuffed animal from my bag.

"Do you think you could help me practice how to change a diaper?" I asked.

Beth laughed. "I don't have kids. I have no clue how to change a diaper," she said.

I wasn't upset because she didn't know how to change a diaper. If you don't have kids and you don't spend time with kids, you don't need to know how to change a diaper—that's fine. What upset me was that she was so dismissive about it. Beth could've asked someone else who did have kids and did know how to change a diaper to help me out. She could've said "You know, I am not the best person to work with you on that, but let me go talk to one of the other therapists and see if they can help."

Beth had no idea how important this was to me. I had two little boys in diapers at home, and I wanted to be doing everything I possibly could be doing to take care of them. I wasn't going to be able to watch them by myself for any great length of time if I couldn't change their diapers. Landon would be out of diapers soon, but Parker still would not be ready to potty train for a little while.

While the therapists at the outpatient rehab center genuinely wanted to help me succeed, I don't think they knew how. Most of the patients the therapists at this center worked with were recovering from strokes. The effects of a stroke are similar to the effects of a brain injury, but they are definitely not the same in every aspect of recovery.

I was also at a totally different place in my life than most of these older people. I had very different goals for my recovery. My goals for physical therapy and occupational therapy were not the same as the older patients recovering from strokes. I didn't just need to care for myself, I needed to care for my young children.

When my physical therapist Kristen and I started working on exercises on the floor mats at the new place, Kristen told me to get down on the mats.

I said I couldn't.

"I don't know how, I don't know where to start, can you…"

"Just get on the floor," she said again, cutting me off.

I tried to explain to her that I literally didn't know how to get down on the floor from a standing position. Alright, fine. I thought to myself, and I just did a seat drop, crashing to the floor full force on my bottom.

Kristen seemed satisfied. I felt frustrated. I

wanted to learn how to get from standing to sitting on the floor without crashing down. There was more to it than just "getting on the floor." This wasn't something that was just going to happen, and this wasn't something I was going to be able to figure out on my own. I needed guidance, and I needed to practice.

Several of my therapy sessions here ended in tears. The worst session was one of the balance exercises, which consisted of a kind of obstacle course. Kristen laid out several canes in a row on the ground. She instructed me to step between the canes.

This was crazy. Hadn't she read any of my medical records? I tried to explain that this exercise was not a good idea. I couldn't see the canes. My depth perception was so out of whack that I wasn't going to be able to direct my step between them. My field of vision was expanding, but my peripheral vision was still very limited. I couldn't see.

Coupled with my vision issues, I really wasn't able to walk very far without my walker. I hadn't worked on walking without a walker at UVA. I walked very little without a walker at the previous out-patient rehab center. I used the treadmill and walked between parallel bars, but I always had something to hold on to. Kristen didn't seem to get it and insisted that I do the exercise.

So I did. Sure enough, disaster struck. I staggered across the row of canes, stepping not in-between but on all of the canes. I was crying and clearly having a hard time, and no one seemed to care. I realized then that this might not be the best place for me.

After a month, I stopped going to that outpatient rehab center. I still had a long way to go, but I felt like I wasn't progressing there. They didn't know how to deal with my issues.

At this point, getting better at daily tasks and chores was a matter of practicing what I'd already learned. I did still need help walking though. I still felt very unsteady with the walker, and I still hoped to walk independently one day. Luke and I would have to do some more research to find someone that could help me.

The second time I fell, it was a rainy Saturday afternoon, and Luke had just finished making lunch for me. I slowly made my way through the kitchen towards the dining area with my walker. When I reached the threshold, I concentrated hard on not stepping on the threshold. Whenever I did that, the uneven ground made me lose my balance. When I say I concentrated hard on not stepping on the threshold, I mean I concentrated on my fear of falling because of losing my balance from stepping on the threshold. I did not concentrate on my steps. I lost my balance. I fell backwards, into the glass china cabinet.

As I fell, time seemed to slow. A wave of terror washed over me. One of my worst fears had finally been realized. Every day, I saw the glass cabinets and glass curios, cluttered with arrangements of yet more glass—china vases and crystal bowls and glass figurines. Every day, I walked in terror of falling and breaking everything. Or worse, what if I fell into all of that glass and broke myself? I felt like a bull in a china shop. Navigating through the furniture and narrow hallways was nerve-wracking.

When I fell into the china cabinet, my elbow hit the glass pane, shattering the glass panel of the china cabinet. My body continued to fall straight to the hardwood floor. I lay there shaken and gasping for breath, but unharmed. My elbow was bleeding a little, but that's it. No deep cuts. No broken bones. That was the extent of the damage. I felt terrible about the shattered glass. I couldn't remember ever breaking something that wasn't mine before, but the glass could be replaced.

Debbie was understanding, which didn't

surprise me in the least. A small amount of chaos ensued trying to keep the boys out of all the broken glass while cleaning it up.

That was my worst fall. I was less afraid of falling after that incident with the china cabinet; I had fallen, hard, and I was okay.

Still, it was a huge fear of mine. I did everything I could to avoid falling while still trying to push myself to get better at walking. It was a delicate balance. Looking back, I realize now that I was only able to learn how to fall by falling again.

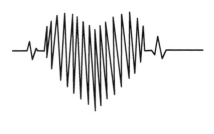

12

In the spring of 2010, Luke and I started causally looking around Ashland for homes. We both agreed that finding a house in Ashland would be best. Even in the best-case scenario of recovery, living close to Mike and Debbie would be essential. Richmond was a half hour drive away from Ashland, longer if there was traffic. If we stayed in Ashland, Mike and Debbie would only be minutes away. With Mike and Debbie so close by, I could try to take care of the boys, again, at small stretches at a time, as I got stronger and better at walking.

We hoped to wait until after spring to move out, so that I could get a little stronger and the boys could get a little more independent, but if the right home came along, we were willing to get things started. And the right home came along: a ranch style handicap accessible home in a great neighborhood, only two miles away from Mike and Debbie's house.

When Luke and I heard about it, we thought it was the answer to our prayers. There was a wheel-chair ramp; the doorways were all very wide; and the bathroom was handicap accessible. The timing wasn't ideal, but both Luke and I saw it as a great opportunity.

Debbie's friend, Anita, lived across the street from the house for-sale. (She's the one that told us about the house.) Anita said a paraplegic man had built the house, which is why it was handicap accessible. The current owner of the house was an elderly woman who needed a wheelchair to get around. She was selling the house because she was about to move to a nursing home. It was just her and her sister, who was taking care of her, living in the house.

The house was a short sale, apparently because it was in no condition to be put on the market. What exactly did that mean? I was a little concerned, but I figured whatever was wrong with it, Luke and our friends and family who had offered their help could fix it.

We went to see the house in March. By then my vision had improved enough that I could see from the car that I didn't think I was interested in this place anymore. My heart sank. I almost told Luke to just keep driving.

It was dirty. It was very dirty. The light grey paint was flaking off everywhere, all of the grass in the lawn was long dead, and the shrubs along the perimeter of the house were in the same state: dead. But maybe it wasn't so bad inside, I told myself.

Andrew, our realtor, stood by the front door waiting for us. He was one of Luke's good friends from high school. He helped us out, free of charge.

After Luke parked the car in the driveway, we all walked around the outside of the property. It was a complete wasteland. Thick, waist high weeds grew over the backyard. The property looked abandoned. Upon closer inspection, I saw that the wheelchair ramp in the garage was too steep, too narrow, and the bend in the middle too sharp for me to navigate. It was not going to work. No way would I be able to wheel myself up there. But that wasn't such a big deal. I was only using my wheelchair when I went out. I used my walker at home. (I hoped to get to the point where I wouldn't need a wheelchair at all. Generally, whenever I came back from being out, rather than unfold the wheelchair to take me the short distance from the garage to the house, Luke walked me in, tightly holding my hand.)

The ramp wasn't a deal breaker, but the inside of the house almost was. When we opened the front door, the first thing we noticed was the smell. Everyone immediately buried their noses in their scarf or shirt collar. Andrew made a strange noise and quietly stepped back outside to stand by the bushes for a few minutes, afraid he was going to be sick. Luke had been to see the house a few days earlier with his dad. His dad didn't even go in the house because he couldn't handle the smell. It was really bad. The smell made being in the house difficult. Walking around inside the house was no easy task either. Boxes, trash, and random pieces of furniture everywhere made moving around difficult. A few narrow pathways had been cleared, and we followed those. It felt like we were hiking in some strange, dark, rank smelling jungle.

Luke was concerned with all of the things that would have to be redone, which was pretty much everything. My concern at the time was the smell. What was it, and where was it coming from?

Looking at the carpets, there had obviously been a lot of cats or dogs here, at some point. It didn't look like any of the animals kept here had ever been let outside to go to the bathroom. I knew from watching countless home improvement shows on HGTV, my favorite channel, that if feces seeped through the carpet down into the sub floor, removing the smell would be very difficult.

It definitely smelled like animals in the worst way, but there was something else that I couldn't put my finger on. There was a stack of dirty adult diapers in the guest bathroom, but that wasn't it. We figured it out when we checked out the kitchen. The fridge was full of rotting, blackened food, crawling with maggots. The smell when we opened the fridge was indescribable. We had to leave after that.

So who would be crazy enough to buy a house that was in such bad shape and smelled so bad? Carolyn and Luke Powell, that's who!

Luke and I were put off by the smell and by how much work the place needed, but the house still met our basic requirements: (1) it was in Ashland; (2) it was one level; and (3) it was big enough for our family. We knew we were going to have a hard time finding a house that met all three of those requirements. The population of Ashland is about 7,000, so there are not a great deal of houses on the market at any given time.

Ashland is an old railroad town. Most of the

houses are old, Dutch colonials, like Mike and Debbie's house. We needed something more spacious. Single story homes with open floor plans are hard to come by around there. Despite the imperfect timing and the condition of the house, we thought that this was a great opportunity.

Buying a house seldom goes according to plan. I used to think the term "short-sale" meant that it would only take a short time to complete the buying process. Not true. "Short-sale" means that the amount of money earned from selling the house falls short of covering what is still owed on the house. It has absolutely nothing to do with time. It was two months before the owners officially accepted our offer, and another month until we could move in. (We had to fix the place up, first.)

If Luke and I bought a house that wasn't handicap accessible, we would have to do a whole lot of work on it anyway. That was our thinking. This house needed even more work than we imagined. We thought we knew what had to be done, but everything ended up dragging out much longer than expected.

Friends, family, and even some of the nurses from the ICU came together to help Luke with the renovations. Together, they ripped out the carpets, treated the floors underneath to get the animal smell out, remodelled the kitchen, knocked out some of the walls in the middle of the house, and gutted the bathrooms. It was a lot of hard work, but I could tell Luke enjoyed wielding a sledgehammer and knocking out the walls and kitchen cabinets.

Once the house was gutted, the renovation team put in new kitchen cabinets, new bathroom fixtures, a new shower, and Brazilian cherry hardwood floors.

One of Luke's best friends since grade school, Erik, helped us with all of the necessary updates. As a contractor, he had a lot of great ideas—like applying a special sealant to the subfloor that is used after a fire in order to keep the animal smells at bay. Erik worked tirelessly on our house until everything was just right.

In place of the wheelchair ramp (which was ripped out), we built a wide platform, like a single, wide stair. This way, I could get down to the garage from the house and back on my own with my walker. The washing machine and dryer were in the garage, so now I could do laundry by myself.

I tested out the platform shortly before we moved in. I felt really good about where I was at. I could do laundry on my own. I could take care of my kids on my own. I could get around this house on my own. There was a light at the end of the tunnel.

This house had a much more open floor plan than Mike and Debbie's house, but I noticed early on that there were some walls in the family room, kitchen, and dining room area that would need to go. Because I couldn't get around very quickly, I wanted to be able to easily see where the kids were at and hear what they were up to. That way, I could make sure they weren't getting into anything they shouldn't be. No matter what kinds of precautions parents try to take, kids—especially young kids—always seem to get into things they shouldn't.

Parker was 18 months old, and Landon was three years old when we moved into our new house. It was inevitable that they would get into stuff. Landon loved to unroll entire toilet paper rolls and climb around on the counters. Like lots of kids his age, Landon had recently taken to removing all of the pots and pans out of the kitchen cabinets. I swear, he could have all the kitchen cabinets emptied in a matter of sixty seconds. I couldn't get to them as quickly as I once could. The sooner I knew that Landon and Parker were getting into trouble, the quicker I could get to them to keep them out of harm's way.

Everyone worked hard, and it just drove me crazy that I couldn't help. I remember watching Luke and his sister, Cara, tear out the old carpets and stopping myself every few minutes from asking, "Hey, can I help?"

Throughout my life, the one thing that always really upset me was being side-lined. That's why Slade and I started off on the wrong foot, because she wouldn't let me play. I wanted to participate. I really love projects like this, and I wanted to take part.

At our house in Richmond, I put up all the curtains, assembled the light fixtures, and painted all the rooms. Between Luke and me, I've always been the handy one around the house. I remember being pregnant with Parker and putting a new backsplash in our kitchen, not because Luke wasn't around, but because I wanted to (and I could).

After three months of hard work, the house was ready. With Landon's help, I unpacked the clothes and put them away in drawers and closets. Even at the age of three, Landon was already turning into my little helper man. Luke purposely left the clothes on the hangers so I would have an easier time putting them away.

The small town feel of Ashland was growing on me. Besides the sparrows and the wrens in the trees, the early hours of the morning were quiet and still. Every morning before breakfast, the boys pressed their noses up against the window in the living room to watch the deer grazing in our front yard. I was amazed by how tame the deer were. In their excitement, Landon and Parker tapped loudly on the windowpane, but the deer never ran off. Much to the boys' delight, the deer instead turned their heads and gazed directly at Landon and Parker.

Mike and Debbie's house had been very full of love and helping hands, but it wasn't a great environment for me to practice walking again. I felt timid, afraid I was going to break something or get hurt. I had nightmares about falling and knocking over one piece of furniture that would knock over another and another, like dominos. I was afraid of knocking over a glass vase and then falling into the glass—or worse, one of the boys getting into the broken glass before I could stop them.

We brought a lot of Landon's and Parker's toys with us to Mike and Debbie's. The only downside was that there was no place for them—no toy boxes, no shelf space. The toys cluttered the house up, and most of the toys just stayed on the floor. I hate clutter. I disliked clutter even more at that time because it made it difficult for me to get around.

This was one of the reasons I was so excited to have our own place again.

Of course, part of the reason I was so timid to practice walking was my fear of falling. I felt stuck. I knew I needed to practice if I was ever going to start walking on my own, but I had a hard time getting past my fear.

By March, Luke and I finally found a therapist to help me out with walking. I knew I liked him from the start. His name was Jeff, and he reminded me a little of Slade in his no-nonsense approach. He got me to push myself. He was very adamant from the beginning that if I wanted to walk on my own without a walker, I was going to have to challenge myself. I was going to have to work through my fear of falling.

In the first week of attending the walking clinic, Jeff said "Carolyn, if you keep using your walker, you're going to be using your walker forever. You're not going to learn how to walk without a walker by using a walker. You're going to learn how to walk without a walker by walking without a walker." He was very much an advocate for patients playing an active role in their own recovery.

I think another reason Jeff was able to get through to me was that he's done a lot of work with athletes. He's coached a lot of teams and served on the U.S. Olympic Committee Medical Team at the Paralympic Games in Atlanta in 1996. I'm not really an athlete anymore, but I was for a long time, right up until the day my heart stopped. So athlete mentality is part of who I am.

Jeff broke down the walking process into parts for me. Walking isn't about just putting one foot in front of the other. Jeff broke down each of the movements and the weight shifts involved. No one had done this for me before. I knew in an abstract way that I would walk again early on in my recovery, but now, with Jeff's help, the prospect of walking on my own became a reality.

Jeff helped me become aware of what my hips, knees, ankles, and feet were doing to make me walk. Paying attention to subtle body movements wasn't entirely new to me. In field hockey, we had to practice correctly shifting our hips. Shifting your hips just the right way as you swing your hockey stick is essential to get the most powerful shot.

Jeff could see that my gait was off; I wasn't correctly shifting my hips. A big part of walking—just like slamming the ball—is correctly shifting your weight by shifting your hips. I was amazed at how easily Jeff detected such subtle variations in my movements. I think the main goal at the rehab hospital was to get me up and moving. I was up and moving forward, just not the right way.

Jeff wanted to start from scratch. Back to the parallel bars to work on balance again. I felt a little discouraged, but it made sense. Jeff assured me that this time around, things would move much faster. My body was much stronger now than it was when I first started trying to use the walker back in Charlottesville.

He was right. This time around, I progressed much more quickly.

In order to walk properly, I needed to push my hips much farther to the sides than I was at that time. When I started at the walking clinic, I still felt wobbly on my feet. When I went to take a step and pushed my hips to the side, I felt like I was going to fall before I pushed them far enough. Even though I felt unstable, I was actually in no real danger of falling. I needed to retrain my brain. The only way that my brain would relearn when I should and when I shouldn't feel unsteady was by pushing myself to the point where I fell.

Jeff took the time to understand me and my individual needs. I think that's one of the reasons that I felt like I could trust him. I didn't entirely believe him when he said "push your hips further to the side, you're not going to fall," but I believed him enough to try. He understood where I was coming from, and if he was convinced that I had it in me to walk again unaided, then so did I.

At the rehab hospital in Charlottesville and the outpatient rehab center in Richmond, I think most of my physical therapists tended to treat me like someone learning to walk after a stroke. A brain injury like mine is similar to a stroke, but it's not the same thing. I don't think stroke survivors experience quite the same disconnect between their brain and their muscles as I did.

When some of the local newspapers ran stories about my recovery, the headline typically read some variation of "Dietician Recovers from Stroke." During the interviews, I never said I had experienced a stroke. I think once I said that I experienced stroke-like symptoms when I was recovering, and they just latched on to that.

Friends and other people I talked to about my experience did the same thing. When I told people that my heart stopped, they said oh, so you had a heart attack. It made me feel like people weren't listening to me. I didn't have a heart attack; my heart went into cardiac arrest.

It was frustrating, but I knew it wasn't really a matter of people not listening or not caring, even though that's what it felt like. It was a matter of trying to understand a complicated situation. Most people are familiar with what a stroke is and what it's like to recover from a stroke. Having a relative or knowing someone who has had a stroke is common, so it's something most people can relate to. People were just trying to understand and relate to my experience. Saying that I have brain damage resulting from my brain being deprived of oxygen because my heart stopped leaves a lot of questions open to individual interpretation.

After six months at the walking clinic, I moved on from balance exercises to start working on walking again. Gripping the bars, I took a step. I made sure my hips shifted correctly. I pushed my hands further down the bars, and I took another step, all the while making sure my hips shifted correctly with each step. My hands always stayed in contact with the bars.

As I became more comfortable, I gradually loosened my grip on the bars. As months passed, I stopped holding on to the bars. My hands hovered just above the bars, ready to grab on should I lose my balance, but I stopped holding on.

Whenever I tried to look up and in front of me while I walked, I felt dizzy and off balance. I needed to see exactly what my feet were doing, and I needed to concentrate on each step if I wanted to maintain my balance. That, and since my peripheral vision was still not very good, I needed to look down to see if there was anything I might trip on, like uneven ground, a door frame, or toy trains.

When I started walking without my walker, I kept my feet far apart and waddled. This wide stance made me feel like I would be able to better maintain my balance. Over the years my stance narrowed somewhat. I don't quite look like a goalie all the time when I'm walking anymore, but it's still a pretty wide stance.

Standing or walking without my walker or the parallel bars, I felt very vulnerable. I felt alone and far out to sea, no land in sight. When I took my first steps, I asked Jeff to hold on to the back of my t-shirt. It made me feel a little better, knowing someone was right there to catch me if I started to fall.

Just as I anticipated, Parker took his first steps while I practiced walking in therapy at the walking clinic. Parker started walking in April, around his first birthday. I was walking with the walker, not on my own just yet. I wasn't able to walk beside him, but I was still able to help him in the beginning. That was huge for me. After missing out on so many of Parker's milestones, I was there for this.

Debbie and I sat on the floor in the living room, about three feet apart. Parker practiced walking from Debbie to me and back. I couldn't lift him up, but when he toddled over to me I gave him a big hug. It wasn't perfect, but motherhood is never perfect. It's all about adapting.

I was already adapting, figuring out new ways to do the things I needed to do to take care of Landon and Parker on my own. I went to therapy at the walking clinic three days a week, the same three days that Landon and Parker now attended preschool.

On the other two days of the week that I didn't go to the walking clinic, I took care of the boys on my own for about an hour before Luke's mom came to pick them up. Having made many failed attempts at bottle feeding and diaper changing, I knew caring for them on my own was going to be a huge challenge, but I looked forward to it.

The first two things I needed to figure out were how to change a diaper (yes – I still had not mastered that) and how to feed the boys. In therapy,

I had a really tough time trying to get the diaper on the stuffed duck. I decided to try using pull-ups in hopes that they would be easier to get on. Pull-ups were much easier than diapers to deal with, but it still wasn't easy. Not by a long shot. There was a lot of preparation involved.

Before I changed Parker, I had to have absolutely everything laid out: a blanket, baby wipes, diaper rash cream, and the pull-up. I had to take out all the baby wipes I thought I would need from the box and have them at the ready. Taking them out of the box while Parker waited to be changed took too much time. I had to do that part before.

The most challenging part about dressing myself was figuring out the difference between the front and the back of my clothes. Pull-ups were no different. The picture on the front of the pull-ups, usually a Disney cartoon character, helped. Without that picture, I wouldn't have known which side of the pull-ups was the front and which side was the back. While the picture on the front helped, I still had to figure out where the leg holes and the waistband were. I would set out the pull-up the same way each time, and pick it up the same way each time.

The easiest way for me to get the new pull-up

on Parker was to sit him on my lap. It was easier for me to stay oriented that way. The slightest change in routine threw me off. Needless to say, I decided to potty train Parker as soon as he turned two. Much to my relief, he caught on quickly and was totally potty trained in a month. What a champ!

I knew even before either Landon or Parker were born that I wanted to steer clear of pre-packaged foods as much as possible. After all, I was a dietician. But our circumstances had been very much altered. I opted for the healthiest single serving pre-packaged food and snacks I could find, like fruit cups, cereal bars, yogurt, and cheese crackers.

One afternoon when Landon and Parker were home from preschool, Landon asked "Hey mom, can I have peanut butter and jelly for lunch. We never have peanut butter and jelly anymore. How come we don't have peanut butter and jelly anymore?"

I'd tried making peanut butter and jelly sandwiches once before, shortly after we moved into the new house in Ashland. It was an epic failure. But I had made a lot of progress in the past couple months. What kind of mother couldn't make her kids a simple peanut butter and jelly sandwich?

The first obstacle was the twist tie on the bag of bread. Could I seriously not get a twist tie off of a bag of bread? Nope. My hands were still too clumsy, and my vision was still too scrambled.

Screw it, I thought and ripped open the side of the bag with my teeth. *Now we're in business.*

I successfully opened the jar of peanut butter and the squeeze bottle of jelly. After that, I'm not really sure what happened. I spread the peanut butter and jelly around, but not very much actually got on the bread. Most of the peanut butter and the jelly was smeared all over the counter.

The aftermath in the kitchen was unbelievable. Comically absurd. It looked like Landon, three years old—not his adult mother—had been making sandwiches. The situation was so ridiculous, that I didn't even feel bad. I just laughed (much like the time I tried to cook a frozen pizza for dinner and put it in the oven with the cardboard underneath).

Once I managed to assemble something that resembled a peanut butter sandwich, I began to put things away. As I was putting the jelly back in the fridge, my hand, slippery and sticky with peanut butter and jelly, slipped off the refrigerator door handle, and bam! I was down on the floor in seconds. The boys were, of course, playing with their trains and blocks on the other side of the room and remained totally oblivious to my chaos.

I managed to pull myself up by holding on to the edge of the counter, somehow managing to get more peanut butter and jelly all over the place. I set the sandwich on a plate on the little kids table that Landon and Parker ate at. It was much easier than me hoisting them up into the kitchen chairs.

Landon sat down and started crying, "Mommy there's crust! I don't LIKE the crust!" I sat down next to him and started pulling bits of crust off with my fingers.

From then on, we started buying the pre-made peanut butter and jelly sandwiches. I always swore to myself I would make my kids lunches, and I would not be one of those people who fed their kids pre-packaged peanut butter sandwiches, and now I swear by them.

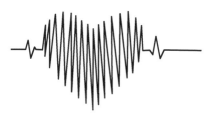

13

With a little creativity and planning, I was changing Parker's pull-ups and preparing lunch for the boys not long after Luke and I moved into our house in Ashland. But I wanted to be doing more. I was eager for the boys to grow up a little.

People say to cherish those early years of a child's life. They pass so fast, people say. But as Parker and Landon grew, they were able to do more for themselves—feed themselves, dress themselves, and use the bathroom by themselves. The more they grew and the more independent they became, the easier it became for me to care for them. But I still wanted to enjoy these precious years when they were young and be a part of their lives as much as I possibly could.

I've always loved giving the boys baths every evening. Luke had taken over that job. He'd taken over a lot of things. Slowly, I tried to do more and more to take care of the boys and help around the house.

A month after we had moved into the house in Ashland, I felt like I was ready to try giving the boys their evening bath. There's no way I would have been able to bathe them myself just a few months earlier. But now, they were bigger and stronger. They could sit up in the tub and get in and out mostly on their own. They were ready, and I was ready. I knew it was going to be a challenge, just like everything else had been. But I didn't anticipate just how mentally, physically, and emotionally difficult bathing two toddler boys would be.

Like absolutely every chore, activity, or task I did, I had to plan out exactly what things I would need beforehand. I had to plan out the order in which I was going to do things. As always, Luke reminded me of all of the steps involved. Just like I didn't remember how to walk, pick up a slice of pizza, or actually do pretty much anything, I didn't fully remember how to give my kids a bath. After Luke patiently described all the steps involved, I felt like I had a good idea of what to do. It wasn't so hard to develop a plan: fill up the tub with water, use the back of my hand to make sure the water was the right temperature, shampoo their heads, wash their bodies with soap, rinse them off, get them out, and dry them off.

But with my handicaps and the boys being so young and unpredictable, I knew I needed to take special care to keep them safe. I had to account for every possible situation. I would need to let the water drain out completely before I got them out of the tub. That way, I could dry them off while they were still sitting in the tub. Drying them off after they were out would've been too difficult. They would be slippery, wet. This way, there was much less of a chance that they would slip.

What would I do if Parker fell and hit his head on the side of the tub? What if Landon got shampoo in his eyes? What if they ate the bathtub crayons? What if Parker slipped back into the water, and I didn't notice in time, and he drowned?

I wanted to be ready for anything, so I played out all kinds of bath-time-gone-horribly-wrong scenarios in my head. I think going through this kind of role playing in my mind was helpful for making sure they were safe, but sometimes my thoughts got out of control. Sometimes I couldn't get my brain to stop creating bath-time catastrophes, most of them ridiculous. By the time I did bathe them for the first time, I was wrecked with anxiety.

I knew I needed to bathe them separately. Bathing them separately would take a little longer, but bathing them together was going to be too much for me. One slippery, squirming little boy would be hard enough to handle—two would be nearly impossible. They were much wilder when they were together. I found that keeping things simple—doing one thing at a time and reducing distractions—was essential. My brain could only handle so much external stimuli. Things needed to be linear. I'm still like this today.

Aside from the pump shampoo bottle, which lots of able-bodied people use, nothing was noticeably different about the kids' bathroom—nothing to suggest their mother had any kind of disability. Several handicap devices, like my walker and shower chair, make things easier for me. But most of my disabilities cannot be overcome by devices alone. There are no devices that can make bathing my children easier—nothing that can help my lack of coordination, muscle weakness, or visual deficits.

For bath time, I laid out towels and pajamas at the ready for Landon and Parker. I could no longer lift Landon into the tub, but I didn't need to. Landon could get in and out of the tub himself. So could Parker. Even still, I held both of their arms tight whenever they got in or out.

The first few bath times were not easy. I had always used a cup to pour water over Landon's head to wet his hair. Those first few times, he squirmed all over the place, and I kept missing his head. And the more I missed, the more he squirmed.

The very first time that I gave Landon a bath, my thighs felt like they were on fire. I went to rest my elbows on the edge of the bathtub, to give my leg muscles a break for a few minutes. Unfortunately, I misjudged the distance and ended up in the water, my sleeves soaking wet. I wanted to cry. Landon played with his little plastic tugboats, oblivious.

Why did this have to be so difficult? Instead of crying, I eased myself out of the water and rolled up my soaking wet sleeves. I decided that from now on, I'd wear short sleeves for bath time. I kept going after I fell into the water, but I wasn't able to finish giving Landon his bath that time. The pain in my thighs became unbearable, and I was completely out of energy. After I washed Landon's hair, Luke had to pick me up off the bathroom floor and carry me to the couch to rest.

Lying there on the couch with my sopping wet sleeves, I felt a lot of different emotions. I felt disappointed, overwhelmed, and proud—but mostly proud. With just a little more stamina, I would be giving Landon and Parker their baths, just like I always had before the cardiac arrest.

When I went over all of the possible scenarios that could unfold during bath-time, I anticipated that bathing the boys was going to be physically challenging for me. I was probably going to get very tired, and I was probably going to be a little sore. But I didn't anticipate just how tired and sore I was going to get.

It had been just over a year after I was admitted to the hospital, and my muscles were still very weak. Just kneeling over the bath felt like deep knee lunges. That was the hardest part. It wasn't just that first time bathing them that my thigh muscles burned; for almost a year, it was every time. I hadn't accounted for this intense pain. I had run through so many scenarios in my head, but this wasn't one of them. I felt overwhelmed by this unaccounted for variable, but I was determined to work past the pain. And, I figured, this had to be great exercise for me.

"Look up at the sky" is what I tell Landon and Parker when I need to wet their hair in the bathtub. And they always do. They listen. Well, almost always.

They might not always listen if I'm telling them

to stop jumping on the couch, but they do listen when it's important. I don't think they know how important this is to me. They don't know how important it is for them either, for their safety. If they are playing too close to the street, I can't just run over and scoop them up like I used to be able to. I have to tell them what to do. I have to tell them to get away from the road, and they do. I tell them to look both ways when we cross the street, and they do. I can hear oncoming cars, but I can't see them well. I can't hold their hands when we cross the street, so I tell them to hold on to my walker, and they do. When I call their names, they always answer immediately. They've always been good about that.

As a result of my impaired vision, my hearing had become very sensitive. This started happening early on, back when I was in the rehabilitation hospital. I noticed I could hear the doctors and nurses whispering about me to each other outside my room. Sometimes I called them out, shouting, "You know I can hear you, right?" once they'd finished talking. I couldn't see them, but by listening to the tone of their voices, I could tell they were probably shaking their heads in amazement.

This increase in the sensitivity of my hearing

helped compensate for my visual impairment in a lot of ways. It was especially helpful in watching the boys. By the time I was caring for them in our house in Ashland, my vision had improved a little, but it was far from perfect. I couldn't see them clearly from one side of the room to the next, and I also couldn't move quickly. I learned to anticipate events and minor calamities by listening closely. If I heard chairs moving across the hardwood floor in the kitchen, I knew Landon was about to climb up on top of the counters. As soon as I heard the chairs on the floor, I started heading over to the kitchen with my walker. Landon wouldn't listen to me telling him to get down while he climbed up the counters. But once he was up and I asked him to put his arms around my neck, so I could safely get him back down, he listened.

I was nervous to let the boys run around outside at first, but I gradually learned to trust both my acute hearing and the boys' listening skills. I didn't want my handicaps to negatively affect Landon and Parker. I wanted them to be able to do the things that kids love doing, like playing outside.

The boys loved running around outside in the yard. They especially loved tooling around the yard in their Power Wheels®. They each got one from Dee-Dee and Pop-Pop that first Christmas that I came home from the hospital. Landon's was a John Deere® Gator Power Wheels®, and Parker had a Jeep® Power Wheels®. It took a few months for Parker to be able to reach the pedals on his own.

On sunny days, I would sit on a wicker bench in the side yard and take in the action. I loved being out there with them, feeling the sunshine on my skin and listening to them play, but I always wished I could be running around with them. That was one of the reasons I had been eager to be a young mother. I wanted to have the energy to keep up with my kids. I wanted to be able to better connect with them, to be a "cool mom."

Now, I had to use a walker to get around. I was still young, and I was still a mother, but I didn't feel like a young mother at all. I felt like an old lady, a grandmother.

Sometimes, when they were riding around in their Power Wheels®, they came across something in the yard or on the edge of the woods that would catch their attention, and they would hop out and explore. If they were more than fifteen feet away, I couldn't see them well. But as long as I could hear either the Power Wheels®, their shouting, or crunching of the leaves under their feet, I knew where they were in the yard.

Whenever they stopped making any noise, I would call out their names, "Landon and Parker?"

They always answered. They still do. That meant as much to me as the bouquets of dandelions and little handfuls of pebbles that they brought back to me from their adventures. As they were explaining what they were up to—"Mommy we found buried treasure!" or "Mommy we're building a trap!"—I was able to hear where they were and shift my gaze around the yard until I found them again.

Both Landon and Parker don't entirely understand what's wrong with me. Landon sometimes asks how I hurt my leg. I tell him that mommy's heart was sick, and it made mommy's brain sick, so she has trouble walking. This seems to satisfy his curiosity for the moment, but I don't think he fully understands. Yet, they understand the importance of listening to me. It's like on some level, they know I cannot see well and that I cannot move fast, so they listen.

With their listening skills and my planning skills, taking care of Landon and Parker went pretty smoothly. Some days, of course, were harder than others. Some days there were tantrums and messes. I'm not the most patient mother in the world, but I don't usually get genuinely upset easily. It happened more often in the first couple years of my recovery.

One Sunday, Luke and I invited some of our friends over to watch the football game, the Washington Redskins v. the Dallas Cowboys. One couple brought their kids over, so Parker and Landon had some playmates for the evening.

Just before half time, I heard giggles coming from Parker and Landon's room. Mischievous sounding giggles. I could tell that the giggles were coming from behind a closed door. Their door was usually open, precisely because I needed to be able to hear what they were up to.

I grabbed my walker and made my way from the couch towards the boys' room. I opened the door to find an epic blanket fort filled with giggling boys. The beds were pushed closer together, and their comforters, sheets and pillows were strewn everywhere.

"Out! Out! Everyone get out!" I shouted.

With wide, downcast eyes, Parker, Landon, and their friends quietly shuffled out of the room. They could tell Mommy was mad. In the doorway of the empty room, holding my walker in front of me, I stood there, surveying the damage.

Two minutes later, my sister-in-law Cara came

to see what all the shouting was about. She found me collapsed in a heap on the sagging blanket fort, sobbing. I had been trying in vain to get one of the sheets back on Landon's bed. I could barely make a bed that was only a little rustled from sleep. Like folding towels, making beds was one of the tasks that I had given up trying to learn for the time being.

How was I going to tackle this mess? And this wasn't going to be the only time my boys made big messes. How was I supposed to keep up with them?

"Hey Carolyn, what's going on?" Cara asked, totally bewildered.

"I have no idea how I am going to clean up this mess…I…I don't even know where to start," I told her. Half laughing, she assured me it was okay.

"I'll help you, it's fine! We'll have this all cleaned up in ten minutes, no problem," she said.

She set to work remaking the beds, her movements smooth and easy—effortless. Making a bed had never been hard for her. I ached for the days when making a bed was easy, when it wasn't something I had to consciously think about. After arranging Parker's pillows on his bed, Cara looked over at me. I was still crying.

"Carolyn, why are you so sad? It's no big deal, we're almost done," she said.

But it was a big deal. It was the first time I realized that I needed help. There were things I was always going to need help with. I hated that I needed help to do things that were so simple. I felt like I had very little control over my own life.

Cara didn't understand why I was so upset. How could she? That was another reason why I was so upset that Sunday afternoon—I realized no one really understood what it was like having to relearn how to do everything. No one realized how difficult and overwhelming seemingly simple tasks were for me. I had to put in a great deal of physical and mental energy to accomplish things that came so natural to everyone else – like making a bed. Even with Cara there, arranging pillows, smoothing blankets, and putting away toys, I felt completely alone.

I felt alone in more ways than one. Living so far from the south side of Richmond, it wasn't easy for friends and family to keep visiting. As time went on, the time between when I saw them was greater and greater. Less than a year after we moved into our house in Ashland, I was alone most days. I had come to feel like a prisoner in my own home, cut off from the rest of the world. I could get around the house okay, but I couldn't drive. My vision was never going to be good enough for me to drive. Most likely, I was going to have to rely on others to get around for the rest of my life. I wanted to move back to the south side of Richmond, closer to my friends. I would be able to see them more often there, and they would be able to give me rides.

Feeling isolated can be a problem for a lot of stay-at-home moms. But this was extreme. I couldn't drive, so I couldn't leave the house, not even to run to the grocery store or the park with the kids to get out of the house. There wasn't really anything within walking distance for me from our home in Ashland. There weren't any kids in our neighborhood either, so Landon and Parker didn't have anyone else to play with when they were at the house. They were still very young, so it wasn't a problem at the time, but later on that was definitely going to be an issue.

As much as I loved spending time with Landon and Parker, and as much as I loved talking about dinosaurs and the finer points of Thomas the Tank Engine with them, I needed social interaction with adults.

Never had I been this miserable before. Despite all the set-backs and obstacles and life changes I'd faced recovering, I never really experienced any feelings of intense sadness or loss. From the beginning of my recovery, I had been working towards a goal—to get back to being a mommy to Landon and Parker—and I was determined to do just that. I felt so happy to have achieved that goal. I felt grateful that I'd been given a second chance. But being so isolated made me absolutely miserable, eclipsing most of that joy.

I felt depressed for a couple of months, but I couldn't really put my finger on why. At first I chalked it up to all of the recent life changes. One day, in the early afternoon when the house was empty, it dawned on me that this was not the life I wanted to be living. Luke was at work, and the boys were both at preschool. I was seated in my big comfy chair in front of the TV, watching who knows what. This is what I did when the house was empty, which was often: sit and watch TV. I've always been a very social person. I had no one to talk to during the day, and I couldn't even get out of the house.

So that evening when Luke came home from work and I told him that I thought we should move back to the south side of Richmond, I was shocked when he said "No way."

I tried giving him reasons why moving back to the south side would be a good idea for both me and our family: My friends and my mother would all be close by, so I could spend more time with them. They could more easily give the boys and me rides. The neighborhood that I had grown up in would be especially ideal—there was a pediatrician, a day care, and a fitness center with a play place for kids all within a short walking distance.

Even after I outlined all of the positive attributes of the south side, his answer remained the same: "No way."

Luke is a very low-key, go with the flow type of guy. Throughout our marriage, I typically got my way—until I brought up moving back to Richmond. We weren't going to move, he said. He put his foot down. We had only lived in our house in Ashland for less than a year. Could I at least just give it some more time?

I was disappointed by his reaction, but I thought maybe he just needed a little time to warm up to the idea. And maybe it wasn't the best time to have brought it up—Luke had been home from work for less than an hour and was trying to make dinner as the boys ran around the kitchen.

If Luke really understood how miserable I was, I knew that he would want to help me. But he didn't understand.

The Heart to Survive

Luke knew I hadn't been in the best of spirits, but I don't think he realized how serious it was. No matter how many times I told him how miserable I felt and that I felt like I was trapped, I just wasn't getting through to him.

Luke and I were more in love than ever before. We were best friends. I knew we were going to get through this rough patch, but I didn't know how.

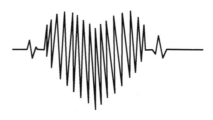

14

Luke was actually the one who suggested we see a counselor together. When he brought it up, I thought it was a great idea. We both knew that a neutral, outside party could help us put things into perspective. Our marriage was great and we loved each other more than ever, but we were having trouble getting past this.

From the first session, I knew we made the right decision.

The room was dimly lit. The furniture, walls, and carpet were all soft blues and earth tones. Besides a little Zen sand garden and a box of tissues on an end table, the room was uncluttered. Our counselor, Samantha, wore her long curly brown hair swept back in a loose braid.

We spent most of the first two sessions laying the groundwork—telling Samantha about ourselves and giving her a general sense of what our relationship was like. I told her all about what I'd been through—the sudden cardiac arrest, the three weeks in the ICU followed by the three months recovering in the rehab hospital, and my struggle to relearn so many things. She was great at getting to the heart of the matter. I think maybe that's one of the reasons I felt like she understood me—we were both people who didn't sugar coat the truth. Early on, I felt like Samantha really understood me as a person and where I was coming from.

During the third session, we got down to business. Luke explained his side of the story, and I explained mine. Samantha asked us each to explain why exactly we were here seeking counseling. I explained how I'd been feeling depressed and isolated. I told her all the reasons why I thought moving back to the south side of Richmond would give me a better quality of life and help me overcome these feelings I'd been struggling with.

"We're here," I said, "because Luke and I are at a standstill. He doesn't think that moving is a good idea. He doesn't think moving is going to really make me happy, but I believe in my heart that it's exactly what I need. Our marriage is great otherwise. I love Luke, and he loves me, but, we're just stuck on this one thing," I explained.

Then it was Luke's turn: "Carolyn is unhappy," Luke said to Samantha. His eyes were solemn. He seldom spoke with so much conviction.

"I want to do whatever it takes for her to get through this, but I don't know what that is. Carolyn really thinks that moving is going to make everything better for her, but I don't think it's the solution. I don't think we should move. We need to be close to my parents, in case she needs help or something happens."

Samantha nodded, and then paused. She put down her clipboard and pen and looked at Luke. "Listen," she said to Luke, "you get to go out and do things. She doesn't. She can't. She doesn't ever get to go out and do things, she's stuck at home. This is her life now, and something needs to change."

That was the moment of clarity for Luke. I'd been saying much the same thing to him for months, but hearing it from someone else made all the difference. It was more real. That third session was a great session—I felt validated, and Luke felt like he understood what I was feeling more. We both felt like a workable solution was just around the corner.

After that conversation, Luke was more willing

to move, but our issues were more complicated than Luke just not having the desire to move. Luke knew I needed a change. He understood why I wanted to move back to the south side of Richmond, but that didn't resolve the two big issues that Luke had with us moving. For one, Luke felt guilty about leaving our house in Ashland. His good friends had poured so much of their own time and effort into helping us fix up the place. They turned a house that was literally rotting into a beautiful home, a home where I was able to be as independent as possible.

The second issue Luke had was a little trickier to reconcile with moving: he wanted us to still be close to his parents. Luke worked long hours and traveled for work frequently. When we started going to counseling in April of 2012, I was strong enough and stable enough to be caring for the boys on my own most of the time. But I still had major handicaps, and Luke wanted to know that either of his parents would be close in case I needed help. Sure, I had a lot of friends and my own mom who all lived in the neighborhood where I wanted to move, but they all had jobs. Luke's mom was at home much of the day. Luke and I both knew some sort of compromise was in order, but we were at a loss as to what that compromise looked like.

When we explained these issues, Samantha suggested we look into moving into a community neighborhood—a neighborhood with a community center and a park within the neighborhood. Neither of us had thought of that as an option before. It sounded like a good compromise. We could try to find a community neighborhood within a 15 minute drive of Luke's parents' house. That way, I could have more of a life, and we'd still be close to his parents.

The next day, Luke and I picked out two neighborhoods with community centers and started house hunting. Both neighborhoods were in Hanover, not far from Ashland. When we decided to buy our house in Ashland, we hadn't given a second thought to the neighborhood. Our main priority was finding somewhere that was handicap accessible and close to Mike and Debbie. This time around, the neighborhood was our top priority. I moved around our house relatively easily now. When we first moved in and I still had major mobility issues, the open floor plan helped me get around more easily and hear what the boys were up to more easily.

But the open floor plan also meant that there was nowhere for me to go to seek refuge from the chaos. After my brain injury, my hearing got sharper and became more sensitive, and my brain was generally more sensitive to external stimuli. I quickly became overwhelmed and anxious when there was too much going on around me. I needed a quiet space where I could go to recharge.

Our only other criteria, besides being in a community neighborhood, were that the house be on a cul-de-sac and have a basement. Those two things weren't deal breakers, but they were important. The basement would give the boys a place to play and be loud and Luke a place to have his friends over to watch football where I wouldn't be able to hear everything. A cul-de-sac meant less traffic, and that meant a safer place for Parker and Landon to play.

Luke started to get excited when we began looking at houses. He realized that this new home could be our forever home. We had both hoped that our home in Ashland was going to be our forever home, but things had changed. Our new home could be a place that better fit our entire family's needs. At our fourth session, after we'd started looking at houses, Samantha was pleasantly surprised at how great we were doing and how much progress we'd made.

The second house we looked at was the one. We loved the neighborhood immediately. As we drove through the neighborhood to the house, families on bicycles waved as we passed, and the playground was crawling with kids. Even more kids played in yards, bouncing and laughing on trampolines and playing tag underneath the big shady trees that had been planted there long before any of the houses.

The house, light brown with blue shutters, was a short walk from the community center and the pool. It was on a cul-de-sac, and it had a huge finished basement. Luke loved the basement, and so did I. A shallow creek ran through the back yard. It was perfect—a perfect place for the boys to grow up, a perfect place for Luke, and a perfect place for me. We moved in to our new home in June of 2012.

Our neighbors say we are meant to be here in Hanover. I could tell when we first came to look at the house that the neighborhood was full of families with kids and that there was a sense of community, but there was no way to know for sure what our neighbors would be like. When you move somewhere, it's hard to get an idea of what your neighbors are like until after you've already moved in.

We were welcomed with open arms and homemade vanilla cupcakes. Many of our neighbors stopped by to personally welcome us into the neighborhood. Some of them brought index cards listing the names of their kids and their home and cell phone numbers. We were invited to frequent block parties — BBQ's or bonfires (depending on the season) in the middle of the cul-de-sac. The neighborhood kids all played basketball out there too – they still do.

Landon and Parker made fast friends with the kids at their new school and in the neighborhood. One neighbor drives Parker to preschool three days a week. Every morning, when I walk Landon to the bus stop, I chat with the other moms waiting with their kids. Seriously, we couldn't have asked for better neighbors.

Needing to rely more on others and learning to accept the help that I need has made me much more aware of my own place in my community. In most neighborhoods in this country, people keep to themselves. That's how most of the neighborhoods I lived in growing up and as an adult were. I love being part of such a close-knit community now.

Our neighbors have been incredibly accepting and helpful to me. Some of them even have kids or close relatives that are handicapped, so they understand where I'm coming from.

When people see a woman in her early thirties using a walker, they are naturally curious. I know I stand out. I stick in people's minds as the young woman with the walker. I think a lot of people assume I have MS. People can be afraid to ask questions, so I try to be upfront. I have no reservations about telling people my story, but it's a long and complicated story.

What I typically tell people when I'm explaining my handicaps is this: I was born with a genetic heart condition called Long QT Syndrome, which can cause sudden cardiac arrest. Two months after my youngest son was born, my heart stopped. My husband found me after checking on my oldest son, who was crying in the middle of the night. My husband did CPR on me until the paramedics arrived. I spent the next three weeks in the ICU and then three months in a rehab hospital, relearning everything: how to walk, how to dress myself, how to eat, how to write—absolutely everything.

Even this explanation leaves a lot out. There isn't a single label that I can use to quickly explain to people why I can't drive to meet them, why I can't read, or why I use a walker. There's not a single medical condition that sums up my handicaps.

The effects of an anoxic brain injury are not easily

described in a nice, succinct yet comprehensive way. The effects vary so much depending on the individual and the amount of time their brain was without oxygen, so saying I had an anoxic brain injury doesn't give anyone a very good idea of my issues. That, and few people are familiar with the term "anoxic brain injury."

Most people I encounter want to help me and want to understand me, but some really don't know how. Sometimes, when Luke and I go to restaurants, servers won't acknowledge me. It was worse when I still used my wheelchair when we went out with the kids. Servers would look at Luke and ask him what I wanted.

"Does she want a water to start off with?" they'd say.

When people like this saw the wheelchair or the walker, they only saw my disability. They didn't see me. I was somehow less of a capable human being. Some people assumed there was something mentally wrong with me, and they didn't know how to deal with it. Maybe people were afraid of offending me, but I would have rather people say something to me—anything—than ignore me. Feeling invisible is one of the most heart-breaking things, for me. It hurts.

The first time I felt ignored like this, Luke and I

were shopping for a new phone for me. I was in my wheelchair at the time. The sales person approached us, but completely ignored me and addressed only Luke. Luke told him I needed a new phone.

Still looking only at Luke, the salesman asked, "What kind of phone does she want?"

Immediately, I shot back with "Hey, are you asking me if I want a new phone? Because I'm right here."

The salesman was taken aback. I don't think he really realized what he had done. "I'm so sorry ma'am. That was rude of me. What kind of phone do you want?"

I don't think he ever made that mistake again. To be fair to the salesmen, I think I was probably looking down.

During the first year that I was home from the rehab hospital, I had a tendency to keep my head down in public. My vision was so bad during that time that I had a hard time figuring out if people were looking directly at me. I thought that if I looked down, people would say my name to get my attention if they wanted to talk to me. If they said my name, then I would know they were talking to me.

After a few incidents of being completely ignored, I started to be more outspoken in the beginning of social interactions. I continued to not make eye contact right away, but I was vocal so people knew I was there and wanted to be part of the conversation.

Landon and Parker were very young when my heart stopped beating. I might have missed out on precious time with my little ones, but I'm grateful they were too young to understand what was going on. They still struggle to understand my handicaps. As I mentioned earlier, they think I've hurt my legs. Parker constantly asks when I'm going to be able to drive and jump. He cannot fathom why I can't jump on a trampoline. But they are getting there. Landon doesn't ask many questions anymore.

Landon and Parker know something is wrong with me. They know I'm not like other mommies. I am not looking forward to the day when they start resenting me because I can't do the things other mommies can do. I only hope that this will be a short-lived phase. I worry that kids at school will make fun of them, but I think I've raised them to be strong and to do the right thing. I make a point to talk to each of them every night. I ask them, "Is everything going okay on the bus? Are people being nice to you at school?"

I tell Landon and Parker that if they are ever

unsure about something or are having problems, they can come to me. "Mommy won't be mad. Mommy will always love you no matter what," I tell them.

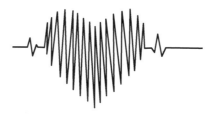

15

Last week, we took the boys to their first pediatric cardiology appointment. Long QT Syndrome can be genetic, so I worry that I may have passed it on to Landon and Parker. So far, the news is good: besides a slight heart murmur, their EKG's and tests came back completely normal.

No sign of Long QT.

However, mine wasn't detected until I was nineteen.

They're not out of the woods yet.

Inherited Long QT Syndrome can remain undetectable until well into adulthood. Until they have the genetic testing done, Landon and Parker will make annual visits to the pediatric cardiologist. We'll avoid giving them certain medications believed to cause dangerous arrhythmias in people who have Long QT, such as certain decongestants and antibiotics. That's really all we can do right now.

Looking back, I can hardly believe how far I have come. In a few months, it will be five years since my cardiac arrest. On the tough days, I try to remind myself how much I've overcome. Some days I get frustrated that I may never be able to work again. There are days when I miss the fast pace of my old life very much. But, there's a lot I'm grateful for.

Within the past year, I finally figured out this crazy puzzle that my life became almost five years ago. A lot of adaptations, some of them major, and some of them not so major, helped me adjust to my physical limitations. My eyeliner is tattooed on—I hate not wearing any make-up, and I still don't have the dexterity in my hands or the vision to put it on myself. I type with one finger at a time, hunting and pecking, as some people say. I have tried various talk-to-text programs, but they are mostly inaccurate and usually a huge hassle. Hunting and pecking is easier. My hands are still very weak and uncoordinated, so I often use my teeth to open packages of food—just as I did to make the first PB&J for Landon and Parker, after my return home from rehab. Most things take me much longer to do than they used to, but I'm just glad I can do them.

The boys are both in school now and doing a lot on their own.

Landon is reading, so he can help me read mail and hand-outs that come home from school when Luke isn't around. Landon also helps Parker, who is just learning to read. I'm walking on my own at home and only using my walker when I go out. I can walk Landon to the bus stop now and wait for the school bus with him.

I still can remember watching Luke's mom walk Landon to preschool while I sat in the car not so very long ago and how badly I wanted to be the one walking Landon to preschool. I've never liked being on the side-lines. Not in field hockey and not in everyday life.

The first time I walked Landon to his preschool class was a warm September day in 2011, over two years after my cardiac arrest. Luke normally dropped Landon off at preschool on his way to work, but he was out of town on business for a few days. Debbie was going to take Landon herself, but I decided to go with her and take the opportunity to walk him to class. She drove and I tagged along.

I had never been to Landon's preschool before, and Landon was beside himself with excitement. He just couldn't wait to show me his classroom. As we walked down the corridor to his class, Landon kept running ahead of me, and I had to keep telling him to slow down.

"Landon, wait for mommy," I kept telling him.

It was slow going, walking with my walker from the car to the building and down the corridor to his classroom, but I felt so proud. I was just as excited as Landon. This was exactly what I had worked so hard in therapy for—getting to be a part of my kids' lives. I remember it all so vividly—that strangely comforting smell of Lysol, crayons, and pencil shavings; the bright colors of all the posters and kids' artwork tacked up on the walls.

Landon opened the door to his classroom, and his teachers warmly greeted both of us. "Good morning Landon! Good morning Mrs. Powell!" they said.

I beamed. The tour began. Landon hung up his backpack and breathlessly ushered me over to his cubby, showing me where all of his things belonged. Then he took me over to the class weather map. There were laminated suns and clouds made out of colored construction paper tacked on to the map each day to reflect the day's weather.

"Mommy, today is sunny, so the sun goes on the map," Landon informed me, holding up the yellow paper sun for me to see.

When Parker starts kindergarten this fall, both boys will be in school. They're not babies anymore. They're growing up and spreading their wings. I'm so grateful that I've been able to raise Landon and Parker and guide them during their most formative years, teaching them right from wrong, the importance of saying please and thank you, and how to communicate. I am so proud of them. They are respectful, helpful, and (most of the time) well mannered. When I see Landon and Parker helping each other zip up their jackets, I know why I worked so hard in therapy. I feel like I've given them a solid foundation.

When I fall, Landon and Parker always rush over to help me. Landon asks if he needs to call 911 or go get help. If I tell them, "Mommy is okay, you don't need to call 911," they give me hugs and kisses. Landon and Parker help me; they help their friends; they help Luke; and most importantly, they help each other.

"He's your only brother, you have to take care of each other," I tell each of them.

They are good kids. I hope I'll be here to watch them grow to adulthood and beyond, but if I'm not, if something happens, I feel confident that they'll be okay without me. They have a good foundation, and they have each other.

My health is good now, but my health was good before my heart stopped. I would've never thought that this would be my life. Life is fragile, things can change in an instant.

Shortly after I came home from the rehab hospital, a high school friend of mine, Tara (my friend who I thought was wearing lingerie when she came to visit and I was still delirious from all the medication I was on), gave me a very special gift: a silver plated bracelet, engraved with a message that really resonated with me. I couldn't read it myself, so Luke read it to me: "Embrace the Journey." It hit home immediately. I had so many challenges ahead of me, so many things to relearn, but I was still here. I needed to get over feeling embarrassed about having a wheelchair and a walker, and I needed to get over being self-conscious about my handicaps and just deal with it.

Luke and I got matching tattoos of that very phrase, Embrace the Journey. When I was in the ICU, Luke promised me that if I made it through, we could get matching tattoos. He definitely had never wanted a tattoo until then. We hadn't decided on what we wanted tattooed until Tara gave me that bracelet. Immediately, we knew that phrase was it. Both Luke and I each have "Embrace the Journey" tattooed on our shoulders.

It took some time, but I've learned to embrace this journey. I've learned to embrace the lack of destination. I won't ever be a hundred percent again, but even now I'm still improving.

There's a lot of uncertainty around brain injuries, but with that uncertainty comes possibility. Relearning how to do walk, take care of myself, and take care of my kids all over again has been an incredible journey. It's been a journey wrought with struggles and triumphs, tears and laughter, frustration and gratitude. It's a journey that I now embrace.

About Carolyn Powell...

Life seemed perfect until early July, when Carolyn's heart stopped due to a heart condition called Long QT Syndrome. She spent the next 4 months in Intensive Care and in a rehabilitation hospital, relearning everything.

Born in Florence, Alabama, in 1981, Carolyn moved to Richmond, Virginia, with her family when she was 7. Carolyn graduated from James River High School in 2000. After high school, Carolyn registered to attend college at James Madison University in Harrisonburg, Virginia.

In the summer of 2001, Carolyn met Luke Powell while waiting tables with him at a restaurant in the Outer Banks of North Carolina. Carolyn graduated from James Madison University in 2004, with her Bachelor of Sciences degree in Dietetics. She married Luke that same summer. Carolyn completed her dietetic internship at the University of Virginia to become a Registered Dietician during the following year.

After Carolyn's internship concluded, Luke and Carolyn moved back to Richmond, near both of their families. Carolyn landed her dream job as the dietician at the University of Richmond. In

August, 2007, Landon was born. Parker followed in April of 2009 – not long after.

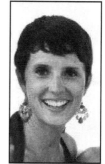

Carolyn now spends most of her time at home, caring for Landon and Parker as a full-time mom. Occasionally, she writes books and blogs about the challenges of her recovery, living with Long QT, and – her favorite topic – parenting her two sons.

Inspired by her children's response to her own disability, Carolyn Powell also published "*Mommy, What is That For?*" A look into the lives of people with disabilities through the eyes of two little boys, this book is a way for parents and teachers to introduce children to certain devices like a walker, wheelchair, braces, and many others. Available now in an ebook format at Barnes and Noble and Amazon!

"*The Heart to Survive*" shares Carolyn's story of survival. Inspiring and uplifting, Carolyn's memoir details how she fought not only to overcome physical hurdles, but also her determination to follow the desires of her heart.

Follow Carolyn on her blog at *www.theheartto-survive.com.*

Shannon Merillat

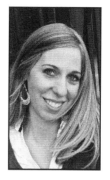

Born in central Florida, Shannon Merillat grew up near the Twin Cities and attended college at St. Olaf College in Northfield, Minnesota, where she received her Bachelor of Arts in English. Shannon completed her graduate degree in Library and Information Studies at the University of Alabama. In addition to freelance ghost-writing projects, Shannon has published poetry and academic articles. In 2013, Shannon presented her research on knowledge sharing at the 2013 Technology, Knowledge, and society Conference in Vancouver, Canada. Shannon currently resides among the rolling hills of England.

Referenced

Munsch, Robert N, and **Sheila McGraw.**
Love You Forever. Scarborough, Ont: Firefly Books, 1986. Print.

Taylor, Jill B.
My Stroke of Insight: A Brain Scientist's Personal Journey. New York: Viking, 2008. Print.